GETTING OFF COCAINE

30 DAYS TO FREEDOM

The Step-by-Step Program of Nutrition and Exercise

GETTING OFF COCAINE

30 DAYS TO FREEDOM

The Step-by-Step Program of Nutrition and Exercise

Michael Weiner, M.S., M.A., Ph.D

COCAINE is a dangerous drug. Withdrawal may also be dangerous. This book is not meant to treat acute cocaine poisoning which can be fatal in minutes; nor is this book made to replace the services of your own physician who should be consulted before you take any medication or treatment.

AVON
PUBLISHERS OF BARD, CAMELOT, DISCUS AND FLARE BOOKS

AVON BOOKS
A division of
The Hearst Corporation
1790 Broadway
New York, New York 10019

Published by arrangement with Quantum Books
Library of Congress Catalog Card Number: 83-25869
ISBN: 0-380-67900-0

Library of Congress Cataloging in Publication Data

Weiner, Michael A.
Getting off cocaine.

Includes bibliographical references.
1. Cocaine habit—Treatment. 2. Cocaine habit—Treatment—Nutritional aspects. 3. Exercise therapy.
I. Title.
RC568.C6W45 1984 616.86′3 83-25869
ISBN 0-380-67900-0

First Avon Printing, February, 1984

Printed in the U. S. A.

DON 10 9 8 7 6 5 4 3 2 1

Canst thou not minister to a mind diseas'd,
Pluck from the memory a rooted sorrow,
Raze out the written troubles of the brain,
And with some sweet oblivious antidote
Cleanse the stuff'd bosom of that perilous stuff
Which weighs upon the heart?

Macbeth (V. iii. 40-45)

ACKNOWLEDGMENTS

Michael Gerber, M.D., for his immensely knowledgeable neurochemical discussions and Alan Eshelman, M.D., Ph.D., for his analysis of my hypothesis.

TABLE OF CONTENTS

PREFACE: A Personal Tragedy xi
CHAPTER 1: Getting Off Cocaine 1
User or Abuser? 1
How Cocaine Works 1
Brain, Blood, and Oxygen 3
Fire in the Brain 5
How Does Nutrition Work Against Cocainism? 10
Cocainism: *Not* an Illness, a Choice 12
CHAPTER 2: 30 Days to Freedom 15
How to Begin 15
Things You Will Need 15
Day-by-Day Plan 18
CHAPTER 3: How Antioxidants Help Cocainists 71
Free Radicals Generated by Cocaine Use Attack Cells 71
How Antioxidants Scavenge Free Radicals 72
CHAPTER 4: Looking Closely (At the Vitamins, Minerals, Amino Acids, Herbs, and Other Things You Will Use) 73
MULTI-VITAMIN/MINERAL 73
Vitamin A 75
Vitamin C 76
Vitamin E 79
Vitamin B Complex 80
Choline and Lecithin 83
Calcium/Magnesium 84
Selenium 85

THE AMINO ACIDS 85
1-Glutamine 86
1-Phenylalanine 87
1-Tyrosine 88
L-Tryptophan 89
L-Cystine 90
ADRENAL EXTRACT 90
HERBS YOU WILL NEED 91
Passionflower 91
Gotu Kola 93
WHY USE "SUDAFED"? 95

CHAPTER 5: Oxygen, Exercise, and the Benefits of Vitamin E 97
The Vitamin That Likes Oxygen 98
Discovery of Vitamin E 98
Oxygen Against Cocaine 99
How to Tell if You Are Deficient 100
Protective Nutrients 101
"E" Against Stress 103

CHAPTER 6: High Energy Nerve Foods 105
Protein Foods Rich in Phenylalanine 105
How the Right Amino Acids Work to Get You "High" 106
Phenylalanine, Content:
Breads, Cereals, Grains 109–110
Dairy, Eggs, Fish, Meats 110–113
Poultry, Game, Lamb, Pork 113–114
Veal, Vegetables, Nuts, Soups 114–116

APPENDIX 1: Treating An Overdose 117
APPENDIX 2: The Coffee Enema 119
APPENDIX 3: Adulterants in Cocaine 125
APPENDIX 4: Bartko's Brain Hypoxia Studies 131
References 135

Preface

A PERSONAL TRAGEDY

I watched a close friend, "Alan," a wealthy stockbroker, go from bad to worse on the "cocaine treatment" offered by a well-meaning medical doctor with many credentials in internal medicine, a Fifth Avenue office in New York, and a fee of $250 an hour. First, he was put on a "detoxification" program consisting of highly toxic barbiturates. A few weeks (and several thousand dollars) later, he was considered "withdrawn" from cocaine; I felt, though, that the good doctor had withdrawn Alan from life.

After a few more weeks he was put on Valium. To compensate for the anxiety, depression, suicidal thinking, killing fatigue, insomnia, apathy, and just plain sadness, an army of toxic drugs was slowly added to his "treatment".

Today, about 18 months later, Alan is still not using cocaine, and is therefore considered a "success" by the doctor. But the man is a wreck—now from the tranquilizers which he is addicted to. He has lost his fabulous home, his wife has left him, and he flounders from one meaningless position to another.

Unfortunately, Alan's doctor refuses to consider

that there might be a natural, nontoxic approach to the cessation of cocaine abuse—a program that promotes health at the same time that it supports withdrawal.

But such an approach does exist, and this book spells it out in simple, day-by-day steps. Using a combination of ordinary nutrients, this natural withdrawal plan is designed to *repair* damage done to the body through months (even years!) of abuse, to compensate for the specific needs of the cocaine abuser, and to alleviate the most common problems experienced by heavy abusers.

This book explains in detail why each nutrient is required and how it works—*not* just to treat the *symptoms* (like barbiturates and Valium), but to give the abuser the "natural high" they've been seeking, possibly all of their forlorn adult lives.

Research in brain biochemistry has advanced far enough for us to know *where* the cocaine molecule acts and *what* it does. This book draws on these findings to define a program for achieving a permanent, natural "high". When blood flow to the brain is increased through exercise and the cells are flooded with added oxygen and glucose, a sense of well-being unlike any artificial high takes over the mind and body. Moreover, by the use of the correct antioxidant vitamins and minerals in the correct dosages, the free-radical damage done by coke (or freebase) is gradually overcome, while the special amino acids in the program act to make an adrenaline-like substance, naturally, within the body itself!

It is not too late even for my friend Alan, who has already been damaged by the standard barbiturate/Valium/pep-talk treatment. Nor is it too late for those millions of others—perhaps your own relative or friend, possibly yourself—for whom this guidebook may be a life changer.

In addition to helping people who are having trouble getting off cocaine, this program will also be useful for those abusing other "excitants" such as amphetamine, methedrine or like compounds. While the action of these drugs differs slightly from that of cocaine, the nutrients, herbs and other elements of my treatment plan will help get them off and *keep* them off by turning them on to a natural sense of well-being, with all the high energy necessary for these competitive times.

Michael A. Weiner, Ph.D.
San Francisco, California 1983

FIGURE 1

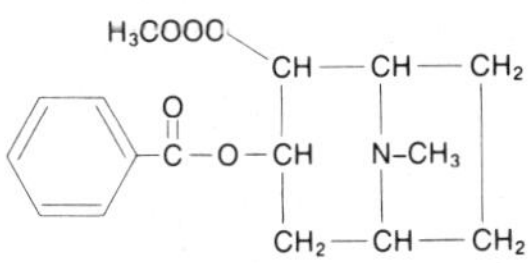

COCAINE

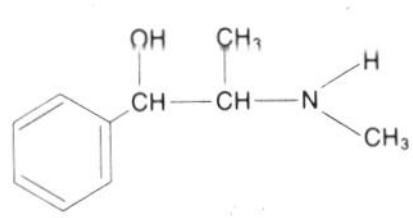

EPHEDRINE
("SUDAFED" is psuedo-ephedrine)

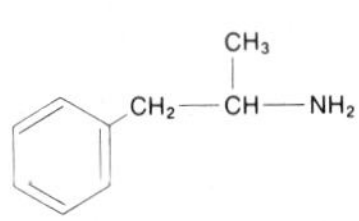

AMPHETAMINE SULFATE
(Benzedrine)

While the chemical structures of cocaine and amphetamine are quite *different* they have very similar pharmacological properties.

TO BEGIN AT ONCE

To begin this program, you can turn to Chapter 2 at once. Then, as you *gradually* add to the treatment plan, one day at a time, day by day for 30 days, you can read through this book at your convenience, to see for yourself why the natural antioxidants, amino acids, vitamins and minerals, and other elements work for you.

A NOTE OF CAUTION

This program is *not* meant to treat *acute* cocaine poisoning, which can be fatal in minutes. Seek *emergency medical care* for a cocaine overdose. Appendix 1 (at the back of this book) is an emergency treatment chart intended only for *physicians* treating acute cocaine poisoning.

After the emergency treatment, upon release from the hospital, this program should work as well as it does for the less severely endangered cocainist.

In addition, the nutritional elements of this program will help relieve specific cocaine withdrawal symptoms, as listed in Table 1—*without* the use of harmful drugs! These withdrawal symptoms, and their natural, nontoxic treatment, are discussed throughout the text.

TABLE 1
COCAINE WITHDRAWAL SYMPTOMS AND SELF TREATMENT INTERVENTIONS*

Symptom	Intervention
Fatigue	Amino acids; adrenal extract; Hypoglycemic diet, rest; coffee enema (optional)
Anxiety	Passionflower herb tea or tincture; vitamin C; choline (a B vitamin)
Depression	Hypoglycemic diet; "Sudafed" (only during initial phase of self treatment); B-complex vitamins; vitamin C
Insomnia	Passionflower herb tea or tincture; tryptophan and magnesium and inositol (a B vitamin)
Hallucinations, delusions, etc.	Niacin (a B vitamin); vitamin C
Muscle aches and twitching	Calcium/magnesium; passionflower herb tea
Weight gain	High protein; high fiber; low carbohydrate diet
Nasal tissue irritation or ulceration (Candida growth in nose)	Herbal ointment (with goldenseal) or vitamin E oil; or aloe vera

**This book is* not *meant to treat* acute *poisoning which can be fatal in minutes. Seek emergency* medical care *for cocaine overdose.*

Chapter 1

GETTING OFF COCAINE

User or Abuser?

Why are some people able to use cocaine occasionally, while others get "addicted"?

Recent research, and a strong framework of neurochemical findings, suggest that the *users* are normal oxygen metabolizers, while *abusers* may be attempting to increase oxygen flow to their brain. Due to *minimal oxygen starvation*, the abuser actually feels "low" all the time—only getting "high" when an oxygen-like rush soothes the needy brain cells.

How Cocaine Works

Cocaine, itself, does not create a "high". The cocaine molecule works by *simulating* the effects of adrenaline-like substances in the nervous system. Here's how.

Nervous signals are carried along the nerves via

electrical and chemical transmitters. In that part of the nervous system where cocaine acts and in all other branches of the nervous system, *chemical transmitters* carry the impulse from one nerve cell to the next.

Do you remember what the end of a nerve cell looks like? You probably saw it in high school biology classes—a sort of long, thin hand with finger-like projections at its end, reaching out toward the fingers of the next nerve. But the two nerves do not quite touch. Between them there is an extremely narrow gap (only 200 Angstroms across—about 2×10^{-5} millimeter).

This gap between nerves is where all the action takes place in the cocaine story. Nerve transmission takes place via chemicals that flow back and forth across this gap, called the *synaptic cleft.*

These natural chemical transmitters flow from one nerve ending to the next and are *recycled,* by flowing back to the first nerve in the sequence. Eventually these chemical transmitters are broken down and the nervous command or impulse is stopped.

Cocaine acts by blocking the recycling of these natural chemical nerve transmitters. By keeping those transmitters there, in the synaptic cleft, an exaggerated hyper-action is triggered. It is as though a switch designed to go "on" and "off" at a rate of about once per second is locked into the "on" mode by cocaine molecules. Instead of a steady, natural nerve transmission we get the well-known, "supercharged" nerve impulse and its attendant effects.

Which explains the "crash" that follows the cocaine "high". By keeping your nervous system "on" with cocaine, you use your available blood sugar and other reserve nutrients for a quick rush. What you are doing is analogous to cashing in your entire bank account for a 20-minute splurge. The analogy is not exact, but conceptually it is accurate. It is as if you have a secure (nutrient) bank balance which you can draw on for 24 hours. But this "balance" requires that you put in a little currency every day, in the form of rest, good nutrition, supplements, and exercise.

By the way, this analogy of cashing in your bank account for a 20-minute splurge works for the *freebase* user as well—only with freebase the "stealing" of your balance is even quicker.

This explanation of how cocaine works at the synapse, between nerves, will be expanded in Chapter 4 when I describe all the nutrients needed to get off coke.

Brain, Blood, and Oxygen

You are walking down a street, absorbed in your latest business deal, love affair, or family problem. Suddenly a car shoots around the corner and comes right at you! For a microsecond you freeze, and then act by jumping out of the way to save yourself.

What happens inside your brain and body during that brief interval can explain the entire cocaine story.

Blood is immediately rushed into your deep muscles so you can run or jump out of the way; simultaneously, a greatly increased amount of blood pours through the carotid arteries into your brain so you can think very sharply and make the right decisions.

But where does this "extra" blood come from? Some is always on reserve, in the spleen and other sites; but during this *emergency demand* the same part of your nervous system that directs extra blood to your brain and deep muscles by *opening up* your blood vessels to these areas (by *dilating* them), also slightly closes off (constricts) the blood vessels going to the peripheral regions of your body. That is why your fingers and toes, your nose and ears become cold during an emergency.

As your body gets ready for "fight or flight", your nervous system transmits different signals via electrical and chemical transmitters. Cocaine works *between* nerves, in the *sympathetic* nervous system, and *mimics* the effects of a real nerve reaction to an emergency situation.

Cocaine is known as a *sympathomimetic* drug because of its ability to mimic a real emergency. That is why it is so popular. That is the *turn-on.* It *excites* people by creating an *adrenaline*-like rush. (Goodman and Gilman, 1970.)

By understanding how cocaine acts we can soon see how the amino acids, vitamins, minerals, foods, and exercise I suggest in the next chapter will act to create a *natural high.*

It's somewhat like the situation with different kinds of sugar. Bear in mind that although a sweet fruit gives you energy, it is *not* the quick energy that you might get from a candy bar. But the fruit gives you *more* than simple energy; it also offers lifesaving food fiber, vitamins, minerals, and some amino acids, plus a host of other *long-acting, age-retarding nutrients.* Sugar will give you a high, but you soon need *more* to get the same "rush". It "speeds you up", but robs you of life-saving nutrients.

Likewise with my program versus cocaine. My program will help you get *off coke* while at the same time *correcting damage* done by cocaine abuse, as well as by the agents used to "cut" coke.* As a bonus, the antioxidants I recommend will scavenge cancer-causing chemical by-products formed from free radicals in the cytochrome system which has been speeded up by cocaine. (Johnson, 1983, Lesser, 1980.)

Before going into the 30-day program you may want to read on a bit further, to comprehend how your craving for cocaine, in its various forms, or for other speed-like activators (such as *amphetamine* or *methedrine*) may be an attempt to dose yourself with a mega quantity of oxygen.

Fire in the Brain

FACT: Your brain accounts for only 3% of your adult body weight, yet demands about 20% of the glucose (blood sugar) required throughout your body.

FACT: One-fifth of all the blood pumped by your heart goes to your brain!

**See Appendix 3 for common adulterants found in cocaine.*

REASON: This organ, wiser than whole rooms of computers, coordinates and integrates all activities of your body. So, it has to be *incessantly active.* It must have a constant supply of *glucose* and *oxygen;* reserves of glucose, glycogen, and ATP (a high-energy bond) can keep it functioning only for minutes, after which *permanent brain damage* will occur.

AND SO: This makes the brain, of all the parts of your body, the most sensitive to a loss of glucose or oxygen. If *either* of these is absent you will *faint* within *seconds,* with *coma* and possibly *death* following in minutes.

Does oxygen consumption increase when cocaine is inhaled, smoked or injected?

We think so. Human experiments have not been possible (for ethical reasons); however, it is known that the cerebral oxygen consumption rate can vary. It is *not a constant,* as once thought.

For example, H.S. Bachelard, Professor of Biochemistry, St. Thomas' Hospital Medical School, London, writes in his book *Brain Biochemistry* (1981): "In epilepsy or induced fits in animals, overall rates of cerebral consumption of glucose and oxygen increase to a considerably greater extent than does the blood flow rate . . . measurements of regional variations in rates of cerebral blood flow have shown changes in specific regions in response to sensory stimuli or mental effort."

Does this prove that cocaine usage increases brain oxygen demands?

As yet, final proof is not possible; but Professor Bachelard describes a new method being used to answer this question more directly. It is based on "the autoradiographic 2-deoxyglucose technique". A radioactive isotope is attached to a portion of the deoxyglucose molecule and "emits positrons which penetrate the skull". This way, the *rate* at which this compound, a sugar, just as glucose, is metabolized within the brain can be monitored.

Using a cyclotron, a "positron emission computed tomography" can tell us the rates at which various regions of the brain are using oxygen and glucose.

Further, stimulants and other drugs which act on the central nervous system (depressants, anesthetics) "may also cause changes in the EEG and in behavior, and in synaptic function, without detectable change in the energy state".

In simpler terms, this means that while we are lacking conclusive proof of increased oxygen demands with cocaine usage, it is known that *oxygen consumption increases* when our *heart rate* increases. Since cocaine increases our pulse, it follows that oxygen consumption also increases.

How does this explain your theory that cocaine abusers may be seeking more oxygen than nonabusers, or abstainers?

Lacking direct, human experimental evidence we must look to experiments conducted with dogs, and to my own clinical experience.

Dr. Daniel Bartko reports on the results of his original research in his book *Experimental Brain Hypoxia* (1971). By cutting off blood flow to the brains of dogs, Dr. Bartko reached several conclusions which lend support to my hypothesis. His results are summarized in Appendix 4, "Brain Hypoxia".

Wait a minute! If the typical cocainist is actually seeking "megadoses of oxygen" via an increased metabolism, why not simply inhale pure oxygen? How come pure oxygen does not result in the same high as you experience with cocaine?

Because oxygen, by itself, is unaccompanied by the increased supply of blood glucose realized when cocaine acts at the synaptic cleft.

Remember, cocaine blocks the reuptake of *noradrenaline*, inhibits the uptake of *serotonin*, prolongs the time *dopamine* acts in the synaptic cleft, inhibits the uptake mechanism of the amino acid precursor *tryptophan*, and inhibits the action of *MAO* (Monoamine oxidase).

Thus, cocaine keeps this system of nervous pathways "on", in an unnatural way.

So, cocaine acts very differently from pure oxygen.

The key to my treatment program is that the balanced, high-protein diet and the amino acids suggested (tryptophan, glutamine, cystine, tyrosine, phenylalanine) will help your body manufacture its own nerve-transmitting chemicals, which act like adrenaline to produce a cocaine-like "high" (but at a more even, sustained level), while at the same time other natural chemicals slow the hyperactive processes initiated by drugs like cocaine and amphetamine, thus producing the smooth rest your overtaxed body and mind require.

What other substances, in addition to oxygen, does cocaine usage create increased demands for?

A significant component of my treatment program calls for increased amounts of certain *amino acids, vitamins,* and *minerals* known to be associated with brain metabolism. It is well known, for example, that vitamin B requirements are greatly increased, owing to the fact that these act as coenzymes in intermediate steps of energy metabolism.

Few doctors have used specific amino acids to act as *excitants.* But some of these amino acids are used by the body to manufacture the important chemical nerve-transmitting substance, noradrenaline. (Bachelard, 1981.)

These include: glutamate, asparate, cystine sulphinate, cysteate, phenylalanine, and tyrosine.

The amino acids, vitamins, minerals, herbs, and other elements of my treatment program are discussed in greater detail in Chapter 4.

At this time we can summarize by stating that the whole body runs on high-energy phosphate bonds, with electrons derived from food combining with oxygen in the cytochrome system in themitochondria, deep within the cells. This fact—that we consume and utilize oxygen for energy—is what distinguishes us from anaerobic bacteria, and is *the essence of our craving for cocaine and other excitants.*

But we pay dearly for having evolved to this high

state—not solely because we constantly crave oxygen, glucose, and other nutrients, but, due to this process of oxygen utilization, we also have to deal with the *toxicity of oxygen!*

This will be detailed later on; for now I simply want to point out that by increasing our metabolism we generate certain free-radical oxygen compounds which must be "quenched" or "scavenged", if we are to prevent these dangerous free radicals from reacting with other molecules in our body and forming new, harmful, sometimes cancer-causing molecules.

When you use cocaine and boost your norepinephrine at the synapse, you push yourself into a higher state of metabolism. Some free radicals are generated from our own metabolic processes, and we must take extra antioxidant nutrients (vitamins A, C, E, and the mineral selenium—discussed in Chapters 3 and 4) to scavenge them. (Johnson, 1982.) This is the debt that we pay for being an oxygen-consuming organism. By using cocaine, we increase this debt enormously.

How Does Nutrition Work Against Cocainism?

Many withdrawal plans exist. Almost all are based on primitive psychological theories which ignore the *physiological* basis of depression, drug seeking, and withdrawal. Cocaine as a chemical is taken to promote sensations thought to be unavailable without the drug. The abuser has typically floundered through a lifetime of "depression", "fatigue", and low self-esteem, and been in and out of therapy. Seldom has a *concentrated,* balanced nutritional approach been utilized to treat the underlying physiological condition which first led to experimentation with cocaine and other euphoriants. Yet, the right foods, vitamins, minerals, amino acids, and herbs, taken in the proper balance, have been employed successfully (to cure even "mental illness") by *enlightened* psychiatrists, physicians, and nutritionists for many years. Much is known about the effects of a lack of certain nutrients and of fluctuating blood sugar on the personality, and tens of thousands of people have been brought back from the nightmare world of depression, self-loathing, even suicidal ideation with *simple dietary changes.* *

With the appearance of this book, I present an integrated, rational program for cocaine withdrawal which utilizes what is known about nutrition and the mind in association with more recent advances in brain chemistry. To treat cocaine addiction, the hypoglycemic diet program** is integrated with other nutrients, supplements, and herbs listed below. All of these together increase blood flow to the brain and hence improve oxygen flow, while also stabilizing blood sugar. In addition, the antioxidant vitamins, minerals, and foods will protect your cells from dangerous free radicals which are the by-product of cocaine usage. Thus, by scavenging these wildly reactive chemical breakdown products (the free radicals), the antioxidant nutrients will prevent membrane penetration and intercept the chemical pathways to many cancers.

**See Fredericks (1969), Kunin (1980), Lesser (1980), Weiner (1981).*

***Each of the above-cited books describes the hypoglycemic disorder and its dietary treatment in great detail, for interested readers.*

Cocainism: *Not* an Illness, a Choice

Using cocaine, freebase, or cocaine paste is psychologically addictive. It may make you think better briefly, grant a moment of euphoria, suppress your desire for food, or act as an aphrodisiac—but the penalties are many. For these moments in heaven there are long hours in the dark corners of hell, where delusions, hallucinations, disorientation, apathy, melancholy, and plain sadness* are constant states, alleviated only by another "blow", "line", or pipeful of smoke.

Despite these harsh pitfalls, millions are willing to pay the price for their few sacred moments of light, where pain, insecurity, doubt, and sadness are nonexistent. With self-perceived benevolence the abusers ride along.

That is *their* business!

The purpose of my book is *not* to preach morality, but to offer an alternative plan for getting "high"—legally and naturally. Obviously, the chronic cynic who prefers the quickness of cocaine to slower methods of ascent will not relate to my nutrition/exercise/supplement regimen—at first. But the day, the hour, the moment will come when he, she or you will be ready to *try anything,* even my legal, natural method.

That is when this book will work.

Willpower is the real fuel for getting off coke.

**These are the psychological symptoms of withdrawal. The physiological picture is uglier—killing fatigue, thrashing insomnia, chills, muscle aches, twitching—all wrapped up in a psychological overlay of guilt, remorse, and thoughts of suicide.*

The nutrients and other supplements and techniques I recommend in my 30-day program will help keep that will *powered!* With a cellular basis of high energy action *and* increased oxygen to the brain *plus* a gradual detoxification using antioxidants to scavenge harmful free radicals (known to incite cell damage, accelerate aging and cancerous reactions), this plan will help the determined determine the course of their own future.

Chapter 2

30 DAYS TO FREEDOM

How to Begin

Try to find all the supplements and other supplies *before you begin "Day 1". But do not* hesitate to initiate the program if you are unable to locate *some* of the items (such as the herbs).

Here is what you will need:

Vitamins and Minerals

Multi Vitamin/Mineral tablets (megadose)*
Vitamin C, 1 gram tablets or capsules or powder
Vitamin E, 100 I.U. capsules
B-Complex, 50 mg. tablets
Calcium/Magnesium tablets (various dosages o.k.)
Choline, 1 gram units
Lecithin, liquid or capsules

**What to look for when buying your multi-formula, as well as each of the other items is discussed in detail in Chapter 4.*

Amino Acids

Phenylalanine capsules, 100 mg.
Glutamine capsules, 100 mg.
Cystine capsules, 500 mg.
Tyrosine capsules, 100 mg.
Tryptophan capsules, 500 mg.

Herbs

Gotu Kola herbal tea (loose)
Passionflower *(Passiflora)* tincture (drops)

Other

"Sudafed" tablets, 30 mg.
Adrenal extract, various brands and potencies
Enema Kits (optional)
Ground coffee (optional)

A Note About Dosages

The dosages suggested are for a 150-pound male without any physical illnesses. You may need more or less of each nutrient depending upon your age, weight, general state of health, and levels of cocaine use.

Pregnant women are cautioned against adopting this program! To withdraw from cocaine or other drugs, see your physician.

THE MIRACLE BODY

The still-miraculous human body is likened to a vast group of buildings in an industrial complex.

To "fix" on a chemical level all the damage done by regular cocaine usage over a long period of time, requires more time, willpower, and an army of nutritional supplements. There is no "instant" answer.

To "feel good" you must first coax your cells and nervous system back to a *normal* operating state; later going *beyond* this state to feel *better* than ever. Vitamins, minerals, amino acids, and an adrenal extract will help replace many of the nutrients lost through spotty eating and little rest. The exercise brings these supplements to your cells more rapidly, increases *oxygen* flow to your brain, and removes toxins more rapidly.

The coffee enema will cleanse your liver which has been severely stressed by metabolizing and detoxifying cocaine and its adulterants. (In the liver, cocaine is hydrolized to ecgonine and benzoyl ecgonine.) However, even though this procedure is simple to perform, and a great catalyzer for the withdrawal program, I call this "optional", since many people are too fastidious to give themselves an enema. Complete instructions for this procedure are found in Appendix 2, "The Coffee Enema".

30 DAYS TO FREEDOM DAY #1

WAKE-UP TIME: Take
☐ 1. Multi Vitamin/Mineral (*Mega* Vitamin Dosage)
☐ 2. Vitamin C, 4 grams
☐ 3. Vitamin E, 100 I.U.
☐ 4. 1 "Sudafed" tablet* (30 mg.)
☐ 5. 1 Phenylalanine capsule, 100 mg.

HALF-WAY THRU: Take
(mid-morning)
☐ 1. Vitamin C, 2 grams
☐ 2. Vitamin E, 100 I.U.

LUNCH (EAT! Even a bit) *Then* take
☐ 1. Phenylalanine capsule, 100 mg.
☐ 2. Vitamin C, 2 grams
☐ 3. 1 "Sudafed" tablet (30 mg.)

ALMOST THRU TIME: Take
☐ 1. Vitamin C, 2 grams
☐ 2. Vitamin E, 100 I.U.
☐ 3. B-Complex, 50–100 mg.

DINNER: (End of stress) Take
☐ 1. Vitamin C, 2 grams
☐ 2. Vitamin E, 100 I.U.
☐ 3. Phenylalanine capsule, 100 mg.

**CAUTION!* "*Sudafed*" *is an over-the-counter pharmaceutical used to relieve allergic symptoms. It is chemically related to ephedrine and similar also to amphetamine. We recommend its use only for those who are not suffering from any of the diseases listed on the side panel of the package. Please read the side panel and follow the precautions. Do Not Exceed One 30 mg. Tablet, 2 times daily. Consult physician if you elect to use longer than 5 days.*

OXYGENATE THRU EXERCISE: 15–20 minutes on the bike, in the pool, a run, brisk walk, dance, chop wood, lift weights or love strongly, even a trampoline.

BEDTIME: Ritually prepare for deep sleep by taking:
☐ 1. 4–6 drops Passiflora in juice
☐ 2. Tryptophan capsules, 1 gram
☐ 3. B-Complex, 50–100 mg.

29 DAYS TO FREEDOM DAY #2

WAKE-UP TIME: Take
☐ 1. Multi Vitamin/Mineral (*Mega* Vitamin Dosage)
☐ 2. Vitamin C, 4 grams
☐ 3. Vitamin E, 100 I.U.
☐ 4. 1 "Sudafed" tablet* (30 mg.)
☐ 5. 1 Phenylalanine capsule, 100 mg.

HALF-WAY THRU: Take
(mid-morning)
☐ 1. Vitamin C, 2 grams
☐ 2. Vitamin E, 100 I.U.

LUNCH (EAT! Even a bit) *Then* take
☐ 1. Phenylalanine capsule, 100 mg.
☐ 2. Vitamin C, 2 grams
☐ 3. 1 "Sudafed" tablet (30 mg.)

ALMOST THRU TIME: Take
☐ 1. Vitamin C, 2 grams
☐ 2. Vitamin E, 100 I.U.
☐ 3. B-Complex, 50–100 mg.

DINNER: (End of stress) Take
☐ 1. Vitamin C, 2 grams
☐ 2. Vitamin E, 100 I.U.
☐ 3. Phenylalanine capsule, 100 mg.

**CAUTION!* *"Sudafed" is an over-the-counter pharmaceutical used to relieve allergic symptoms. It is chemically related to ephedrine and similar also to amphetamine. We recommend its use only for those who are not suffering from any of the diseases listed on the side panel of the package. Please read the side panel and follow the precautions. Do Not Exceed One 30 mg. Tablet, 2 times daily. Consult physician if you elect to use longer than 5 days.*

OXYGENATE THRU EXERCISE: 15–20 minutes on the bike, in the pool, a run, brisk walk, dance, chop wood, lift weights or love strongly, even a trampoline.

BEDTIME: Ritually prepare for deep sleep by taking:
☐ 1. 4–6 drops Passiflora in juice
☐ 2. Tryptophan capsules, 1 gram
☐ 3. B-Complex, 50–100 mg.

28 DAYS TO FREEDOM **DAY #3**

WAKE-UP TIME: Take
☐ 1. Multi Vitamin/Mineral (*Mega* Vitamin Dosage)
☐ 2. Vitamin C, 4 grams
☐ 3. Vitamin E, 100 I.U.
☐ 4. 1 "Sudafed" tablet* (30 mg.)
☐ 5. 1 Phenylalanine capsule, 100 mg.

HALF-WAY THRU: Take
(mid-morning)
☐ 1. Vitamin C, 2 grams
☐ 2. Vitamin E, 100 I.U.

LUNCH (EAT! Even a bit) *Then* take
☐ 1. Phenylalanine capsule, 100 mg.
☐ 2. Vitamin C, 2 grams
☐ 3. 1 "Sudafed" tablet (30 mg.)

ALMOST THRU TIME: Take
☐ 1. Vitamin C, 2 grams
☐ 2. Vitamin E, 100 I.U.
☐ 3. B-Complex, 50–100 mg.

DINNER: (End of stress) Take
☐ 1. Vitamin C, 2 grams
☐ 2. Vitamin E, 100 I.U.
☐ 3. Phenylalanine capsule, 100 mg.

**CAUTION! "Sudafed" is an over-the-counter pharmaceutical used to relieve allergic symptoms. It is chemically related to ephedrine and similar also to amphetamine. We recommend its use only for those who are not suffering from any of the diseases listed on the side panel of the package. Please read the side panel and follow the precautions. Do Not Exceed One 30 mg. Tablet, 2 times daily. Consult physician if you elect to use longer than 5 days.*

OXYGENATE THRU EXERCISE: 15–20 minutes on the bike, in the pool, a run, brisk walk, dance, chop wood, lift weights or love strongly, even a trampoline.

BEDTIME: Ritually prepare for deep sleep by taking:
☐ 1. 4–6 drops Passiflora in juice
☐ 2. Tryptophan capsules, 1 gram
☐ 3. B-Complex, 50–100 mg.

27 DAYS TO FREEDOM DAY #4

WAKE-UP TIME: Take
☐ 1. Tyrosine capsule, 100 mg.
☐ 2. Multi Vitamin/Mineral
☐ 3. Vitamin C, 4 grams
☐ 4. Vitamin E, 100 I.U.
☐ 5. Phenylalanine capsule, 100 mg.

HALF-WAY THRU: Take
(mid-morning)
☐ 1. Vitamin C, 2 grams
☐ 2. Vitamin E, 100 I.U.

LUNCH (EAT! Even a bit) *Then* take
☐ 1. Phenylalanine capsule, 100 mg.
☐ 2. Vitamin C, 2 grams
☐ 3. Calcium/magnesium, 250 mg.

ALMOST THRU TIME: Take
☐ 1. Vitamin C, 2 grams
☐ 2. Vitamin E, 100 I.U.
☐ 3. B-Complex, 50–100 mg.

DINNER: (End of stress) Take
☐ 1. Calcium/magnesium, 250 mg.
☐ 2. Vitamin C, 2 grams
☐ 3. Vitamin E, 100 I.U.
☐ 4. Phenylalanine capsule, 100 mg.

OXYGENATE THRU EXERCISE: 15–20 minutes on the bike, in the pool, a run, brisk walk, dance, chop wood, lift weights or love strongly, even a trampoline.

BEDTIME: Ritually prepare for deep sleep by taking:
☐ 1. Calcium/magnesium, 250 mg.
☐ 2. 4–6 drops Passiflora in juice
☐ 3. Tryptophan capsule, 1 gram
☐ 4. B-Complex, 50–100 mg.

26 DAYS TO FREEDOM **DAY #5**

WAKE-UP TIME: Take
☐ 1. Tyrosine capsule, 100 mg.
☐ 2. Multi Vitamin/Mineral
☐ 3. Vitamin C, 4 grams
☐ 4. Vitamin E, 100 I.U.
☐ 5. Phenylalanine capsule, 100 mg.

HALF-WAY THRU: Take
(mid-morning)
☐ 1. Vitamin C, 2 grams
☐ 2. Vitamin E, 100 I.U.

LUNCH (EAT! Even a bit) *Then* take
☐ 1. Phenylalanine capsule, 100 mg.
☐ 2. Vitamin C, 2 grams
☐ 3. Calcium/magnesium, 250 mg.

ALMOST THRU TIME: Take
☐ 1. Vitamin C, 2 grams
☐ 2. Vitamin E, 100 I.U.
☐ 3. B-Complex, 50–100 mg.

DINNER: (End of stress) Take
☐ 1. Calcium/magnesium, 250 mg
☐ 2. Vitamin C, 2 grams
☐ 3. Vitamin E, 100 I.U.
☐ 4. Phenylalanine capsule, 100 mg.

OXYGENATE THRU EXERCISE: 15–20 minutes on the bike, in the pool, a run, brisk walk, dance, chop wood, lift weights or love strongly, even a trampoline.

BEDTIME: Ritually prepare for deep sleep by taking:
☐ 1. Calcium/magnesium, 250 mg.
☐ 2. 4–6 drops Passiflora in juice
☐ 3. Tryptophan capsule, 1 gram
☐ 4. B-Complex, 50–100 mg.

25 DAYS TO FREEDOM **DAY #6**

WAKE-UP TIME: Take
☐ 1. Tyrosine capsule, 100 mg.
☐ 2. Multi Vitamin/Mineral
☐ 3. Vitamin C, 4 grams
☐ 4. Vitamin E, 100 I.U.
☐ 5. Phenylalanine capsule, 100 mg.

HALF-WAY THRU: Take
(mid-morning)
☐ 1. Vitamin C, 2 grams
☐ 2. Vitamin E, 100 I.U.

LUNCH (EAT! Even a bit) *Then* take
☐ 1. Phenylalanine capsule, 100 mg.
☐ 2. Vitamin C, 2 grams
☐ 3. Calcium/magnesium, 250 mg.

ALMOST THRU TIME: Take
☐ 1. Vitamin C, 2 grams
☐ 2. Vitamin E, 100 I.U.
☐ 3. B-Complex, 50–100 mg.

DINNER: (End of stress) Take
☐ 1. Calcium/magnesium, 250 mg.
☐ 2. Vitamin C, 2 grams
☐ 3. Vitamin E, 100 I.U.
☐ 4. Phenylalanine capsule, 100 mg.

OXYGENATE THRU EXERCISE: 15–20 minutes on the bike, in the pool, a run, brisk walk, dance, chop wood, lift weights or love strongly, even a trampoline.

BEDTIME: Ritually prepare for deep sleep by taking:
☐ 1. Calcium/magnesium, 250 mg.
☐ 2. 4–6 drops Passiflora in juice
☐ 3. Tryptophan capsule, 1 gram
☐ 4. B-Complex, 50–100 mg.

24 DAYS TO FREEDOM — DAY #7

WAKE-UP TIME: Take

☐ 1. 1 cup Gotu Kola herbal tea
☐ 2. Glutamine capsule, 500 mg.
☐ 3. Tyrosine capsule, 100 mg.
☐ 4. Multi Vitamin/Mineral
☐ 5. Vitamin C, 4 grams
☐ 6. Vitamin E, 200 I.U.
☐ 7. Phenylalanine capsule, 200 mg.

HALF-WAY THRU: Take
(mid-morning)

☐ 1. Vitamin C, 2 grams
☐ 2. Vitamin E, 200 I.U.

LUNCH (EAT! Even a bit) *Then* take

☐ 1. Phenylalanine capsule, 100 mg.
☐ 2. Vitamin C, 2 grams
☐ 3. Calcium/magnesium, 250 mg.

ALMOST THRU TIME: Take

☐ 1. Vitamin C, 2 grams
☐ 2. Vitamin E, 200 I.U.
☐ 3. B-Complex, 50–100 mg.
☐ 4. Gotu Kola herbal tea, 1 cup

DINNER: (End of stress) Take

☐ 1. Glutamine capsule, 500 mg.
☐ 2. Calcium/magnesium, 250 mg.
☐ 3. Vitamin C, 2 grams
☐ 4. Vitamin E, 200 I.U.
☐ 5. Phenylalanine capsule, 100 mg.
☐ 6. Coffee enema (Optional, see Appendix 2)

OXYGENATE THRU EXERCISE: 15–20 minutes on the bike, in the pool, a run, brisk walk, dance, chop wood, lift weights or love strongly, even a trampoline.

BEDTIME: Ritually prepare for deep sleep by taking:

☐ 1. Calcium/magnesium, 250 mg.
☐ 2. 4–6 drops Passiflora in juice
☐ 3. Tryptophan capsule, 1 gram
☐ 4. B-Complex, 50–100 mg.

23 DAYS TO FREEDOM DAY #8

WAKE-UP TIME: Take
☐ 1. 1 cup Gotu Kola herbal tea
☐ 2. Glutamine capsule, 500 mg.
☐ 3. Tyrosine capsule, 100 mg.
☐ 4. Multi Vitamin/Mineral
☐ 5. Vitamin C, 4 grams
☐ 6. Vitamin E, 200 I.U.
☐ 7. Phenylalanine capsule, 200 mg.

HALF-WAY THRU: Take
(mid-morning)
☐ 1. Vitamin C, 2 grams
☐ 2. Vitamin E, 200 I.U.

LUNCH (EAT! Even a bit) *Then* take
☐ 1. Phenylalanine capsule, 100 mg.
☐ 2. Vitamin C, 2 grams
☐ 3. Calcium/magnesium, 250 mg.

ALMOST THRU TIME: Take
☐ 1. Vitamin C, 2 grams
☐ 2. Vitamin E, 200 I.U.
☐ 3. B-Complex, 50–100 mg.
☐ 4. Gotu Kola herbal tea, 1 cup

DINNER: (End of stress) Take
☐ 1. Glutamine capsule, 500 mg.
☐ 2. Calcium/magnesium, 250 mg.
☐ 3. Vitamin C, 2 grams
☐ 4. Vitamin E, 200 I.U.
☐ 5. Phenylalanine capsule, 100 mg.
☐ 6. Coffee enema (Optional, see Appendix 2)

OXYGENATE THRU EXERCISE: 15–20 minutes on the bike, in the pool, a run, brisk walk, dance, chop wood, lift weights or love strongly, even a trampoline.

BEDTIME: Ritually prepare for deep sleep by taking:

☐ 1. Calcium/magnesium, 250 mg.
☐ 2. 4–6 drops Passiflora in juice
☐ 3. Tryptophan capsule, 1 gram
☐ 4. B-Complex, 50–100 mg.

22 DAYS TO FREEDOM — DAY #9

WAKE-UP TIME: Take

☐ 1. 1 cup Gotu Kola herbal tea
☐ 2. Glutamine capsule, 500 mg.
☐ 3. Tyrosine capsule, 100 mg.
☐ 4. Multi Vitamin/Mineral
☐ 5. Vitamin C, 4 grams
☐ 6. Vitamin E, 200 I.U.
☐ 7. Phenylalanine capsule, 200 mg.

HALF-WAY THRU: Take
(mid-morning)

☐ 1. Vitamin C, 2 grams
☐ 2. Vitamin E, 200 I.U.

LUNCH (EAT! Even a bit) *Then* take

☐ 1. Phenylalanine capsule, 100 mg.
☐ 2. Vitamin C, 2 grams
☐ 3. Calcium/magnesium, 250 mg.

ALMOST THRU TIME: Take

☐ 1. Vitamin C, 2 grams
☐ 2. Vitamin E, 200 I.U.
☐ 3. B-Complex, 50–100 mg.
☐ 4. Gotu Kola herbal tea, 1 cup

DINNER: (End of stress) Take

☐ 1. Glutamine capsule, 500 mg.
☐ 2. Calcium/magnesium, 250 mg.
☐ 3. Vitamin C, 2 grams
☐ 4. Vitamin E, 200 I.U.
☐ 5. Phenylalanine capsule, 100 mg.
☐ 6. Coffee enema (Optional, see Appendix 2)

OXYGENATE THRU EXERCISE: 15-20 minutes on the bike, in the pool, a run, brisk walk, dance, chop wood, lift weights or love strongly, even a trampoline.

BEDTIME: Ritually prepare for deep sleep by taking:

- ☐ 1. Calcium/magnesium, 250 mg.
- ☐ 2. 4–6 drops Passiflora in juice
- ☐ 3. Tryptophan capsule, 1 gram
- ☐ 4. B-Complex, 50–100 mg.

21 DAYS TO FREEDOM **DAY #10**

WAKE-UP TIME: Take
- ☐ 1. Cystine capsule, 500 mg.
- ☐ 2. Glutamine capsule, 500 mg.
- ☐ 3. Tyrosine capsule, 100 mg.
- ☐ 4. Phenylalanine capsule, 200 mg.
- ☐ 5. Multi Vitamin/Mineral
- ☐ 6. Vitamin C, 4 grams
- ☐ 7. Vitamin E, 200 I.U.
- ☐ 8. Gotu Kola herbal tea, 1 cup

HALF-WAY THRU: Take
(mid-morning)
- ☐ 1. Vitamin C, 2 grams
- ☐ 2. Vitamin E, 200 I.U.

LUNCH (EAT! Even a bit) *Then* Take
- ☐ 1. Cystine capsule, 500 mg.
- ☐ 2. Glutamine capsule, 500 mg.
- ☐ 3. Phenylalanine capsule, 100 mg.
- ☐ 4. Vitamin C, 2 grams
- ☐ 5. Calcium/magnesium, 250 mg.

ALMOST THRU TIME: Take
- ☐ 1. Vitamin C, 2 grams
- ☐ 2. Vitamin E, 200 I.U.
- ☐ 3. B-Complex, 50–100 mg.
- ☐ 4. Gotu Kola herbal tea, 1 cup

DINNER: (End of stress) Take
- ☐ 1. Cystine capsule, 500 mg.
- ☐ 2. Glutamine capsule, 500 mg.
- ☐ 3. Calcium/magnesium, 250 mg.
- ☐ 4. Vitamin C, 2 grams
- ☐ 5. Vitamin E, 200 I.U.
- ☐ 6. Phenylalanine capsule, 100 mg.
- ☐ 7. Coffee enema (Optional, see Appendix 2)

OXYGENATE THRU EXERCISE: 15–20 minutes on the bike, in the pool, a run, brisk walk, dance, chop wood, lift weights or love strongly, even a trampoline.

BEDTIME: Ritually prepare for deep sleep by taking:
☐ 1. Calcium/magnesium, 250 mg.
☐ 2. 4–6 drops Passiflora in juice
☐ 3. Tryptophan capsule, 1 gram
☐ 4. B-Complex, 50–100 mg.

20 DAYS TO FREEDOM **DAY #11**

WAKE-UP TIME: Take
- ☐ 1. Cystine capsule, 500 mg.
- ☐ 2. Glutamine capsule, 500 mg.
- ☐ 3. Tyrosine capsule, 100 mg.
- ☐ 4. Phenylalanine capsule, 200 mg.
- ☐ 5. Multi Vitamin/Mineral
- ☐ 6. Vitamin C, 4 grams
- ☐ 7. Vitamin E, 200 I.U.
- ☐ 8. Gotu Kola herbal tea, 1 cup

HALF-WAY THRU: Take
(mid-morning)
- ☐ 1. Vitamin C, 2 grams
- ☐ 2. Vitamin E, 200 I.U.

LUNCH (EAT! Even a bit) *Then* take
- ☐ 1. Cystine capsule, 500 mg.
- ☐ 2. Glutamine capsule, 500 mg.
- ☐ 3. Phenylalanine capsule, 100 mg.
- ☐ 4. Vitamin C, 2 grams
- ☐ 5. Calcium/magnesium, 250 mg.

ALMOST THRU TIME: Take
- ☐ 1. Vitamin C, 2 grams
- ☐ 2. Vitamin E, 200 I.U.
- ☐ 3. B-Complex, 50–100 mg.
- ☐ 4. Gotu Kola herbal tea, 1 cup

DINNER: (End of stress) Take
- ☐ 1. Cystine capsule, 500 mg.
- ☐ 2. Glutamine capsule, 500 mg.
- ☐ 3. Calcium/magnesium, 250 mg.
- ☐ 4. Vitamin C, 2 grams
- ☐ 5. Vitamin E, 200 I.U.
- ☐ 6. Phenylalanine capsule, 100 mg.
- ☐ 7. Coffee enema (Optional, see Appendix 2)

OXYGENATE THRU EXERCISE: 15–20 minutes on the bike, in the pool, a run, brisk walk, dance, chop wood, lift weights or love strongly, even a trampoline.

BEDTIME: Ritually prepare for deep sleep by taking:
☐ 1. Calcium/magnesium, 250 mg.
☐ 2. 4–6 drops Passiflora in juice
☐ 3. Tryptophan capsule, 1 gram
☐ 4. B-Complex, 50–100 mg.

19 DAYS TO FREEDOM **DAY #12**

WAKE-UP TIME: Take
☐ 1. Cystine capsule, 500 mg.
☐ 2. Glutamine capsule, 500 mg.
☐ 3. Tyrosine capsule, 100 mg.
☐ 4. Phenylalanine capsule, 200 mg.
☐ 5. Multi Vitamin/Mineral
☐ 6. Vitamin C, 4 grams
☐ 7. Vitamin E, 200 I.U.
☐ 8. Gotu Kola herbal tea, 1 cup

HALF-WAY THRU: Take
(mid-morning)
☐ 1. Vitamin C, 2 grams
☐ 2. Vitamin E, 200 I.U.

LUNCH (EAT! Even a bit) *Then* take
☐ 1. Cystine capsule, 500 mg.
☐ 2. Glutamine capsule, 500 mg.
☐ 3. Phenylalanine capsule, 100 mg.
☐ 4. Vitamin C, 2 grams
☐ 5. Calcium/magnesium, 250 mg.

ALMOST THRU TIME: Take
☐ 1. Vitamin C, 2 grams
☐ 2. Vitamin E, 200 I.U.
☐ 3. B-Complex, 50–100 mg.
☐ 4. Gotu Kola herbal tea, 1 cup

DINNER: (End of stress) Take
☐ 1. Cystine capsule, 500 mg.
☐ 2. Glutamine capsule, 500 mg.
☐ 3. Calcium/magnesium, 250 mg.
☐ 4. Vitamin C, 2 grams
☐ 5. Vitamin E, 200 I.U.
☐ 6. Phenylalanine capsule, 100 mg.
☐ 7. Coffee enema (Optional, see Appendix 2)

OXYGENATE THRU EXERCISE: 15–20 minutes on the bike, in the pool, a run, brisk walk, dance, chop wood, lift weights or love strongly, even a trampoline.

BEDTIME: Ritually prepare for deep sleep by taking:

☐ 1. Calcium/magnesium, 250 mg.
☐ 2. 4–6 drops Passiflora in juice
☐ 3. Tryptophan capsule, 1 gram
☐ 4. B-Complex, 50–100 mg.

18 DAYS TO FREEDOM DAY #13

WAKE-UP TIME: Take

☐ 1. Cystine capsule, 500 mg.
☐ 2. Glutamine capsule, 1 gram
☐ 3. Tyrosine capsule, 100 mg.
☐ 4. Phenylalanine capsule, 200 mg.
☐ 5. Multi Vitamin/Mineral
☐ 6. Vitamin C, 4 grams
☐ 7. Vitamin E, 200 I.U.
☐ 8. Gotu Kola herbal tea, 1 cup

HALF-WAY THRU: Take (mid-morning)

☐ 1. Vitamin C, 2 grams
☐ 2. Vitamin E, 200 I.U.
☐ 3. Choline, 1–5 grams
☐ 4. Lecithin, 1–6 tablespoons

LUNCH (EAT! Even a bit) *Then* take

☐ 1. Cystine capsule, 500 mg.
☐ 2. Glutamine capsule, 1 gram
☐ 3. Phenylalanine capsule, 100 mg.
☐ 4. Vitamin C, 2 grams
☐ 5. Calcium/magnesium, 250 mg.

ALMOST THRU TIME: Take

☐ 1. Vitamin C, 2 grams
☐ 2. Vitamin E, 200 I.U.
☐ 3. B-Complex, 50–100 mg.
☐ 4. Gotu Kola herbal tea, 1 cup

DINNER: (End of stress) Take

☐ 1. Cystine capsule, 500 mg.
☐ 2. Glutamine capsule, 1 gram
☐ 3. Calcium/magnesium, 250 mg.
☐ 4. Vitamin C, 2 grams
☐ 5. Vitamin E, 200 I.U.

- ☐ 6. Phenylalanine capsule, 200 mg.
- ☐ 7. Coffee enema (Optional, see Appendix 2)

OXYGENATE THRU EXERCISE: 15–20 minutes on the bike, in the pool, a run, brisk walk, dance, chop wood, lift weights or love strongly, even a trampoline.

BEDTIME: Ritually prepare for deep sleep by taking:

- ☐ 1. Calcium/magnesium, 250 mg.
- ☐ 2. 4–6 drops Passiflora in juice
- ☐ 3. Tryptophan capsule, 1 gram
- ☐ 4. B-Complex, 50–100 mg.

17 DAYS TO FREEDOM **DAY #14**

WAKE-UP TIME: Take
- ☐ 1. Cystine capsule, 500 mg.
- ☐ 2. Glutamine capsule, 1 gram
- ☐ 3. Tyrosine capsule, 100 mg.
- ☐ 4. Phenylalanine capsule, 200 mg.
- ☐ 5. Multi Vitamin/Mineral
- ☐ 6. Vitamin C, 4 grams
- ☐ 7. Vitamin E, 200 I.U.
- ☐ 8. Gotu Kola herbal tea, 1 cup

HALF-WAY THRU: Take
(mid-morning)
- ☐ 1. Vitamin C, 2 grams
- ☐ 2. Vitamin E, 200 I.U.
- ☐ 3. Choline, 1–5 grams
- ☐ 4. Lecithin, 1–6 tablespoons

LUNCH (EAT! Even a bit) *Then* take
- ☐ 1. Cystine capsule, 500 mg.
- ☐ 2. Glutamine capsule, 1 gram
- ☐ 3. Phenylalanine capsule, 100 mg.
- ☐ 4. Vitamin C, 2 grams
- ☐ 5. Calcium/magnesium, 250 mg.

ALMOST THRU TIME: Take
- ☐ 1. Vitamin C, 2 grams
- ☐ 2. Vitamin E, 200 I.U.
- ☐ 3. B-Complex, 50–100 mg.
- ☐ 4. Gotu Kola herbal tea, 1 cup

DINNER. (End of stress) Take
- ☐ 1. Cystine capsule, 500 mg.
- ☐ 2. Glutamine capsule, 1 gram
- ☐ 3. Calcium/magnesium, 250 mg.
- ☐ 4. Vitamin C, 2 grams
- ☐ 5. Vitamin E, 200 I.U.

☐ 6. Phenylalanine capsule, 200 mg.
☐ 7. Coffee enema (Optional, see Appendix 2)

OXYGENATE THRU EXERCISE: 15–20 minutes on the bike, in the pool, a run, brisk walk, dance, chop wood, lift weights or love strongly, even a trampoline.

BEDTIME: Ritually prepare for deep sleep by taking:
☐ 1. Calcium/magnesium, 250 mg.
☐ 2. 4–6 drops Passiflora in juice
☐ 3. Tryptophan capsule, 1 gram
☐ 4. B-Complex, 50–100 mg.

16 DAYS TO FREEDOM DAY #15

WAKE-UP TIME: Take

☐ 1. Cystine capsule, 500 mg.
☐ 2. Glutamine capsule, 1 gram
☐ 3. Tyrosine capsule, 100 mg.
☐ 4. Phenylalanine capsule, 200 mg.
☐ 5. Multi Vitamin/Mineral
☐ 6. Vitamin C, 4 grams
☐ 7. Vitamin E, 200 I.U.
☐ 8. Gotu Kola herbal tea, 1 cup

HALF-WAY THRU: Take
(mid-morning)

☐ 1. Vitamin C, 2 grams
☐ 2. Vitamin E, 200 I.U.
☐ 3. Choline, 1–5 grams
☐ 4. Lecithin, 1–6 tablespoons

LUNCH (EAT! Even a bit) *Then* take

☐ 1. Cystine capsule, 500 mg.
☐ 2. Glutamine capsule, 1 gram
☐ 3. Phenylalanine capsule, 100 mg.
☐ 4. Vitamin C, 2 grams
☐ 5. Calcium/magnesium, 250 mg.

ALMOST THRU TIME: Take

☐ 1. Vitamin C, 2 grams
☐ 2. Vitamin E, 200 I.U.
☐ 3. B-Complex, 50–100 mg.
☐ 4. Gotu Kola herbal tea, 1 cup

DINNER: (End of stress) Take

☐ 1. Cystine capsule, 500 mg.
☐ 2. Glutamine capsule, 1 gram
☐ 3. Calcium/magnesium, 250 mg.
☐ 4. Vitamin C, 2 grams
☐ 5. Vitamin E, 200 I.U.

- ☐ 6. Phenylalanine capsule, 200 mg.
- ☐ 7. Coffee enema (Optional, see Appendix 2)

OXYGENATE THRU EXERCISE: 15–20 minutes on the bike, in the pool, a run, brisk walk, dance, chop wood, lift weights or love strongly, even a trampoline.

BEDTIME: Ritually prepare for deep sleep by taking:

- ☐ 1. Calcium/magnesium, 250 mg.
- ☐ 2. 4–6 drops Passiflora in juice
- ☐ 3. Tryptophan capsule, 1 gram
- ☐ 4. B-Complex, 50–100 mg.

15 DAYS TO FREEDOM DAY #16

HALFWAY POINT!

WAKE-UP TIME: Take
☐ 1. Cystine capsule, 1 gram
☐ 2. Glutamine capsule, 1 gram
☐ 3. Tyrosine capsule, 100 mg.
☐ 4. Phenylalanine capsule, 200 mg.
☐ 5. Multi Vitamin/Mineral
☐ 6. Vitamin C, 4 grams
☐ 7. Vitamin E, 200 I.U.
☐ 8. Gotu Kola herbal tea, 1 cup
☐ 9. Adrenal extract tablet

HALF-WAY THRU: Take
(mid-morning)
☐ 1. Vitamin C, 2 grams
☐ 2. Vitamin E, 200 I.U.
☐ 3. Choline, 1–5 grams
☐ 4. Lecithin, 1–6 tablespoons

LUNCH (EAT! Even a bit) *Then* take
☐ 1. Cystine capsule, 1 gram
☐ 2. Glutamine capsule, 1 gram
☐ 3. Phenylalanine capsule, 100 mg.
☐ 4. Vitamin C, 2 grams
☐ 5. Calcium/magnesium, 250 mg.

ALMOST THRU TIME: Take
☐ 1. Vitamin C, 2 grams
☐ 2. Vitamin E, 200 I.U.
☐ 3. B-Complex, 50–100 mg.
☐ 4. Gotu Kola herbal tea, 1 cup

DINNER: (End of stress) Take
☐ 1. Cystine capsule, 1 gram
☐ 2. Glutamine capsule, 1 gram
☐ 3. Calcium/magnesium, 250 mg.
☐ 4. Vitamin C, 2 grams

- ☐ 5. Vitamin E, 200 I.U.
- ☐ 6. Phenylalanine capsule, 200 mg.
- ☐ 7. Coffee enema (Optional, see Appendix 2)

OXYGENATE THRU EXERCISE: 15–20 minutes on the bike, in the pool, a run, brisk walk, dance, chop wood, lift weights or love strongly, even a trampoline.

BEDTIME: Ritually prepare for deep sleep by taking:

- ☐ 1. Calcium/magnesium, 250 mg.
- ☐ 2. 4–6 drops Passiflora in juice
- ☐ 3. Tryptophan capsule, 1 gram
- ☐ 4. B-Complex, 50–100 mg.

14 DAYS TO FREEDOM DAY #17

WAKE-UP TIME: Take
☐ 1. Cystine capsule, 1 gram
☐ 2. Glutamine capsule, 1 gram
☐ 3. Tyrosine capsule, 100 mg.
☐ 4. Phenylalanine capsule, 200 mg.
☐ 5. Multi Vitamin/Mineral
☐ 6. Vitamin C, 4 grams
☐ 7. Vitamin E, 200 I.U.
☐ 8. Gotu Kola herbal tea, 1 cup
☐ 9. Adrenal extract tablet

HALF-WAY THRU: Take
(mid-morning)
☐ 1. Vitamin C, 2 grams
☐ 2. Vitamin E, 200 I.U.
☐ 3. Choline, 1–5 grams
☐ 4. Lecithin, 1–6 tablespoons

LUNCH (EAT! Even a bit) *Then* take
☐ 1. Cystine capsule, 1 gram
☐ 2. Glutamine capsule, 1 gram
☐ 3. Phenylalanine capsule, 100 mg.
☐ 4. Vitamin C, 2 grams
☐ 5. Calcium/magnesium, 250 mg.

ALMOST THRU TIME: Take
☐ 1. Vitamin C, 2 grams
☐ 2. Vitamin E, 200 I.U.
☐ 3. B-Complex, 50–100 mg.
☐ 4. Gotu Kola herbal tea, 1 cup

DINNER: (End of stress) Take
☐ 1. Cystine capsule, 1 gram
☐ 2. Glutamine capsule, 1 gram
☐ 3. Calcium/magnesium, 250 mg.
☐ 4. Vitamin C, 2 grams
☐ 5. Vitamin E, 200 I.U.

☐ 6. Phenylalanine capsule, 200 mg.
☐ 7. Coffee enema (Optional, see Appendix 2)

OXYGENATE THRU EXERCISE: 15–20 minutes on the bike, in the pool, a run, brisk walk, dance, chop wood, lift weights or love strongly, even a trampoline.

BEDTIME: Ritually prepare for deep sleep by taking:
☐ 1. Calcium/magnesium, 250 mg.
☐ 2. 4–6 drops Passiflora in juice
☐ 3. Tryptophan capsule, 1 gram
☐ 4. B-Complex, 50–100 mg.

13 DAYS TO FREEDOM DAY #18

WAKE-UP TIME: Take
☐ 1. Cystine capsule, 1 gram
☐ 2. Glutamine capsule, 1 gram
☐ 3. Tyrosine capsule, 100 mg.
☐ 4. Phenylalanine capsule, 200 mg.
☐ 5. Multi Vitamin/Mineral
☐ 6. Vitamin C, 4 grams
☐ 7. Vitamin E, 200 I.U.
☐ 8. Gotu Kola herbal tea, 1 cup
☐ 9. Adrenal extract tablet

HALF-WAY THRU: Take
(mid-morning)
☐ 1. Vitamin C, 2 grams
☐ 2. Vitamin E, 200 I.U.
☐ 3. Choline, 1–5 grams
☐ 4. Lecithin, 1–6 tablespoons

LUNCH (EAT! Even a bit) *Then* take
☐ 1. Cystine capsule, 1 gram
☐ 2. Glutamine capsule, 1 gram
☐ 3. Phenylalanine capsule, 100 mg.
☐ 4. Vitamin C, 2 grams
☐ 5. Calcium/magnesium, 250 mg.

ALMOST THRU TIME: Take
☐ 1. Vitamin C, 2 grams
☐ 2. Vitamin E, 200 I.U.
☐ 3. B-Complex, 50–100 mg.
☐ 4. Gotu Kola herbal tea, 1 cup

DINNER: (End of stress) Take
☐ 1. Cystine capsule, 1 gram
☐ 2. Glutamine capsule, 1 gram
☐ 3. Calcium/magnesium, 250 mg.
☐ 4. Vitamin C, 2 grams
☐ 5. Vitamin E, 200 I.U.

☐ 6. Phenylalanine capsule, 200 mg.
☐ 7. Coffee enema (Optional, see Appendix 2)

OXYGENATE THRU EXERCISE: 15–20 minutes on the bike, in the pool, a run, brisk walk, dance, chop wood, lift weights or love strongly, even a trampoline.

BEDTIME: Ritually prepare for deep sleep by taking:
☐ 1. Calcium/magnesium, 250 mg.
☐ 2. 4–6 drops Passiflora in juice
☐ 3. Tryptophan capsule, 1 gram
☐ 4. B-Complex, 50–100 mg.

12 DAYS TO FREEDOM — DAY #19

WAKE-UP TIME: Take
- ☐ 1. Cystine capsule, 1 gram
- ☐ 2. Glutamine capsule, 1 gram
- ☐ 3. Tyrosine capsule, 100 mg.
- ☐ 4. Phenylalanine capsule, 200 mg.
- ☐ 5. Multi Vitamin/Mineral
- ☐ 6. Vitamin C, 4 grams
- ☐ 7. Vitamin E, 200 I.U.
- ☐ 8. Gotu Kola herbal tea, 1 cup
- ☐ 9. Adrenal extract tablet

HALF-WAY THRU: Take
(mid-morning)
- ☐ 1. Vitamin C, 2 grams
- ☐ 2. Vitamin E, 200 I.U.
- ☐ 3. Choline, 1–5 grams
- ☐ 4. Lecithin, 1–6 tablespoons

LUNCH (EAT! Even a bit) *Then* take
- ☐ 1. Cystine capsule, 1 gram
- ☐ 2. Glutamine capsule, 1 gram
- ☐ 3. Phenylalanine capsule, 100 mg.
- ☐ 4. Vitamin C, 2 grams
- ☐ 5. Calcium/magnesium, 250 mg.

ALMOST THRU TIME: Take
- ☐ 1. Vitamin C, 2 grams
- ☐ 2. Vitamin E, 200 I.U.
- ☐ 3. B-Complex, 50–100 mg.
- ☐ 4. Gotu Kola herbal tea, 1 cup

DINNER: (End of stress) Take
- ☐ 1. Cystine capsule, 1 gram
- ☐ 2. Glutamine capsule, 1 gram
- ☐ 3. Calcium/magnesium, 250 mg.
- ☐ 4. Vitamin C, 2 grams
- ☐ 5. Vitamin E, 200 I.U.

☐ 6. Phenylalanine capsule, 200 mg.
☐ 7. Coffee enema (Optional, see Appendix 2)

OXYGENATE THRU EXERCISE: 15–20 minutes on the bike, in the pool, a run, brisk walk, dance, chop wood, lift weights or love strongly, even a trampoline.

BEDTIME: Ritually prepare for deep sleep by taking:
☐ 1. Calcium/magnesium, 250 mg.
☐ 2. 4–6 drops Passiflora in juice
☐ 3. Tryptophan capsule, 1 gram
☐ 4. B-Complex, 50–100 mg.

11 DAYS TO FREEDOM DAY #20

(Note REDUCTIONS in vitamins)

WAKE-UP TIME: Take
☐ 1. Cystine capsule, 1 gram
☐ 2. Glutamine capsule, 1 gram
☐ 3. Tyrosine capsule, 100 mg.
☐ 4. Phenylalanine capsule, 200 mg.
☐ 5. Multi Vitamin/Mineral
☐ 6. Vitamin C, 2–4 grams
☐ 7. Vitamin E, 200 I.U.
☐ 8. Gotu Kola herbal tea, 1 cup
☐ 9. Adrenal extract tablet

HALF-WAY THRU: Take
(mid-morning)
☐ 1. Vitamin C, 1–2 grams
☐ 2. Vitamin E, 200 I.U.
☐ 3. Choline, 1–5 grams
☐ 4. Lecithin, 1–6 tablespoons

LUNCH (EAT! Even a bit) *Then* take
☐ 1. Cystine capsule, 1 gram
☐ 2. Glutamine capsule, 1 gram
☐ 3. Phenylalanine capsule, 100 mg.
☐ 4. Vitamin C, 1–2 grams
☐ 5. Calcium/magnesium, 250 mg.

ALMOST THRU TIME: Take
☐ 1. Vitamin C, 2 grams
☐ 2. Vitamin E, 200 I.U.
☐ 3. B-Complex, 50–100 mg.
☐ 4. Gotu Kola herbal tea, 1 cup

DINNER: (End of stress) Take
☐ 1. Cystine capsule, 1 gram
☐ 2. Glutamine capsule, 1 gram
☐ 3. Calcium/magnesium, 250 mg.
☐ 4. Vitamin C, 1–2 grams

☐ 5. Vitamin E, 200 I.U.
☐ 6. Phenylalanine capsule, 200 mg.
☐ 7. Coffee enema (Optional, see Appendix 2)

OXYGENATE THRU EXERCISE: 15–20 minutes on the bike, in the pool, a run, brisk walk, dance, chop wood, lift weights or love strongly, even a trampoline.

BEDTIME: Ritually prepare for deep sleep by taking:
☐ 1. Calcium/magnesium, 250 mg.
☐ 2. 4–6 drops Passiflora in juice
☐ 3. Tryptophan capsule, 1 gram
☐ 4. B-Complex, 50–100 mg.

10 DAYS TO FREEDOM — DAY #21

WAKE-UP TIME: Take

- ☐ 1. Cystine capsule, 1 gram
- ☐ 2. Glutamine capsule, 1 gram
- ☐ 3. Tyrosine capsule, 100 mg.
- ☐ 4. Phenylalanine capsule, 200 mg.
- ☐ 5. Multi Vitamin/Mineral
- ☐ 6. Vitamin C, 2–4 grams
- ☐ 7. Vitamin E, 200 I.U.
- ☐ 8. Gotu Kola herbal tea, 1 cup
- ☐ 9. Adrenal extract tablet

HALF-WAY THRU: Take
(mid-morning)

- ☐ 1. Vitamin C, 1–2 grams
- ☐ 2. Vitamin E, 200 I.U.
- ☐ 3. Choline, 1–5 grams
- ☐ 4. Lecithin, 1–6 tablespoons

LUNCH (EAT! Even a bit) *Then* Take

- ☐ 1. Cystine capsule, 1 gram
- ☐ 2. Glutamine capsule, 1 gram
- ☐ 3. Phenylalanine capsule, 100 mg.
- ☐ 4. Vitamin C, 1–2 grams
- ☐ 5. Calcium/magnesium, 250 mg.

ALMOST THRU TIME: Take

- ☐ 1. Vitamin C, 2 grams
- ☐ 2. Vitamin E, 200 I.U.
- ☐ 3. B-Complex, 50–100 mg.
- ☐ 4. Gotu Kola herbal tea, 1 cup

DINNER: (End of stress) Take

- ☐ 1. Cystine capsule, 1 gram
- ☐ 2. Glutamine capsule, 1 gram
- ☐ 3. Calcium/magnesium, 250 mg.
- ☐ 4. Vitamin C, 1–2 grams
- ☐ 5. Vitamin E, 200 I.U.

☐ 6. Phenylalanine capsule, 200 mg.
☐ 7. Coffee enema (Optional, see Appendix 2)

OXYGENATE THRU EXERCISE: 15–20 minutes on the bike, in the pool, a run, brisk walk, dance, chop wood, lift weights or love strongly, even a trampoline.

BEDTIME: Ritually prepare for deep sleep by taking:
☐ 1. Calcium/magnesium, 250 mg.
☐ 2. 4–6 drops Passiflora in juice
☐ 3. Tryptophan capsule, 1 gram
☐ 4. B-Complex, 50–100 mg.

9 DAYS TO FREEDOM **DAY #22**

WAKE-UP TIME: Take

☐ 1. Cystine capsule, 1 gram
☐ 2. Glutamine capsule, 1 gram
☐ 3. Tyrosine capsule, 100 mg.
☐ 4. Phenylalanine capsule, 200 mg.
☐ 5. Multi Vitamin/Mineral
☐ 6. Vitamin C, 2–4 grams
☐ 7. Vitamin E, 200 I.U.
☐ 8. Gotu Kola herbal tea, 1 cup
☐ 9. Adrenal extract tablet

HALF-WAY THRU: Take
(mid-morning)

☐ 1. Vitamin C, 1–2 grams
☐ 2. Vitamin E, 200 I.U.
☐ 3. Choline, 1–5 grams
☐ 4. Lecithin, 1–6 tablespoons

LUNCH (EAT! Even a bit) *Then* take

☐ 1. Cystine capsule, 1 gram
☐ 2. Glutamine capsule, 1 gram
☐ 3. Phenylalanine capsule, 100 mg.
☐ 4. Vitamin C, 1–2 grams
☐ 5. Calcium/magnesium, 250 mg.

ALMOST THRU TIME: Take

☐ 1. Vitamin C, 2 grams
☐ 2. Vitamin E, 200 I.U.
☐ 3. B-Complex, 50–100 mg.
☐ 4. Gotu Kola herbal tea, 1 cup

DINNER: (End of stress) Take

☐ 1. Cystine capsule, 1 gram
☐ 2. Glutamine capsule, 1 gram
☐ 3. Calcium/magnesium, 250 mg.
☐ 4. Vitamin C, 1–2 grams
☐ 5. Vitamin E, 200 I.U.

☐ 6. Phenylalanine capsule, 200 mg.
☐ 7. Coffee enema (Optional, see Appendix 2)

OXYGENATE THRU EXERCISE: 15–20 minutes on the bike, in the pool, a run, brisk walk, dance, chop wood, lift weights or love strongly, even a trampoline.

BEDTIME: Ritually prepare for deep sleep by taking:
☐ 1. Calcium/magnesium, 250 mg.
☐ 2. 4–6 drops Passiflora in juice
☐ 3. Tryptophan capsule, 1 gram
☐ 4. B-Complex, 50–100 mg.

8 DAYS TO FREEDOM **DAY #23**

(Note REDUCTIONS in amino acids)

WAKE-UP TIME: Take
- ☐ 1. Cystine capsule, 1 gram
- ☐ 2. Glutamine capsule, 1 gram
- ☐ 3. Tyrosine capsule, 100 mg.
- ☐ 4. Phenylalanine capsule, 200 mg.
- ☐ 5. Multi Vitamin/Mineral
- ☐ 6. Vitamin C, 1–3 grams
- ☐ 7. Vitamin E, 200 I.U.

HALF-WAY THRU: Take
(mid-morning)
- ☐ 1. Vitamin C, 1–2 grams
- ☐ 2. Vitamin E, 200 I.U.
- ☐ 3. Choline, 1–3 grams
- ☐ 4. Lecithin, 1+ tablespoons

LUNCH (EAT! Even a bit) *Then* take
- ☐ 1. Vitamin C, 1–2 grams
- ☐ 2. Calcium/magnesium, 250 mg.

ALMOST THRU TIME: Take
- ☐ 1. B-Complex, 50–100 mg.
- ☐ 2. Gotu Kola herbal tea, 1 cup
- ☐ 3. Vitamin C, 1 gram
- ☐ 4. Vitamin E, 100 I.U.

DINNER: (End of stress) Take
- ☐ 1. Cystine capsule, 1 gram
- ☐ 2. Glutamine capsule, 1 gram
- ☐ 3. Phenylalanine capsule, 200 mg.
- ☐ 4. Vitamin C, 1 gram
- ☐ 5. Vitamin E, 100 I.U.

OXYGENATE THRU EXERCISE: 15–20 minutes on the bike, in the pool, a run, brisk walk, dance, chop wood, lift weights or love strongly, even a trampoline.

BEDTIME: Ritually prepare for deep sleep by taking:

☐ 1. Calcium/magnesium, 250 mg.
☐ 2. 4–6 drops Passiflora in juice
☐ 3. Tryptophan capsule, 1 gram

7 DAYS TO FREEDOM **DAY #24**

ONE WEEK TO GO!

WAKE-UP TIME: Take
- ☐ 1. Cystine capsule, 1 gram
- ☐ 2. Glutamine capsule, 1 gram
- ☐ 3. Tyrosine capsule, 100 mg.
- ☐ 4. Phenylalanine capsule, 200 mg.
- ☐ 5. Multi Vitamin/Mineral
- ☐ 6. Vitamin C, 1–3 grams
- ☐ 7. Vitamin E, 200 I.U.

HALF-WAY THRU: Take (mid-morning)
- ☐ 1. Vitamin C, 1–2 grams
- ☐ 2. Vitamin E, 200 I.U.
- ☐ 3. Choline, 1–3 grams
- ☐ 4. Lecithin, 1+ tablespoons

LUNCH (EAT! Even a bit) *Then* take
- ☐ 1. Vitamin C, 1–2 grams
- ☐ 2. Calcium/magnesium, 250 mg.

ALMOST THRU TIME: Take
- ☐ 1. B-Complex, 50–100 mg.
- ☐ 2. Gotu Kola herbal tea, 1 cup
- ☐ 3. Vitamin C, 1 gram
- ☐ 4. Vitamin E, 100 I.U.

DINNER: (End of stress) Take
- ☐ 1. Cystine capsule, 1 gram
- ☐ 2. Glutamine capsule, 1 gram
- ☐ 3. Phenylalanine capsule, 200 mg.
- ☐ 4. Vitamin C, 1 gram
- ☐ 5. Vitamin E, 100 I.U.

OXYGENATE THRU EXERCISE: 15–20 minutes on the bike, in the pool, a run, brisk walk, dance, chop wood, lift weights or love strongly, even a trampoline.

BEDTIME: Ritually prepare for deep sleep by taking:

☐ 1. Calcium/magnesium, 250 mg.
☐ 2. 4–6 drops Passiflora in juice
☐ 3. Tryptophan capsule, 1 gram

6 DAYS TO FREEDOM **DAY #25**

WAKE-UP TIME: Take
- ☐ 1. Cystine capsule, 1 gram
- ☐ 2. Glutamine capsule, 1 gram
- ☐ 3. Tyrosine capsule, 100 mg.
- ☐ 4. Phenylalanine capsule, 200 mg.
- ☐ 5. Multi Vitamin/Mineral
- ☐ 6. Vitamin C, 1–3 grams
- ☐ 7. Vitamin E, 200 I.U.

HALF-WAY THRU: Take
(mid-morning)
- ☐ 1. Vitamin C, 1–2 grams
- ☐ 2. Vitamin E, 200 I.U.
- ☐ 3. Choline, 1–3 grams
- ☐ 4. Lecithin, 1+ tablespoons

LUNCH (EAT! Even a bit) *Then* take
- ☐ 1. Vitamin C, 1–2 grams
- ☐ 2. Calcium/magnesium, 250 mg.

ALMOST THRU TIME: Take
- ☐ 1. B-Complex, 50–100 mg.
- ☐ 2. Gotu Kola herbal tea, 1 cup
- ☐ 3. Vitamin C, 1 gram
- ☐ 4. Vitamin E, 100 I.U.

DINNER: (End of stress) Take
- ☐ 1. Cystine capsule, 1 gram
- ☐ 2. Glutamine capsule, 1 gram
- ☐ 3. Phenylalanine capsule, 200 mg.
- ☐ 4. Vitamin C, 1 gram
- ☐ 5. Vitamin E, 100 I.U.

OXYGENATE THRU EXERCISE: 15–20 minutes on the bike, in the pool, a run, brisk walk, dance, chop wood, lift weights or love strongly, even a trampoline.

BEDTIME: Ritually prepare for deep sleep by taking:

☐ 1. Calcium/magnesium, 250 mg.
☐ 2. 4–6 drops Passiflora in juice
☐ 3. Tryptophan capsule, 1 gram

5 DAYS TO FREEDOM **DAY #26**

WAKE-UP TIME: Take
- ☐ 1. Multi Vitamin/Mineral
- ☐ 2. Vitamin C, 1 gram
- ☐ 3. Vitamin E, 100 I.U.
- ☐ 4. Phenylalanine (if needed)
- ☐ 5. Gotu Kola herbal tea, 1 cup

HALF-WAY THRU: Take
(mid-morning)
- ☐ 1. Vitamin C, 1 gram
- ☐ 2. Vitamin E, 100 I.U.
- ☐ 3. Choline, 1 gram
- ☐ 4. Lecithin, 1 tablespoon

LUNCH (EAT! Even a bit) *Then* take
- ☐ 1. Vitamin C, 1 gram
- ☐ 2. Calcium/magnesium, 250 mg.

ALMOST THRU TIME: Take
- ☐ 1. B-Complex, 50–100 mg.
- ☐ 2. Vitamin C, 1 gram
- ☐ 3. Vitamin E, 100 I.U.
- ☐ 4. Phenylalanine (if needed)

DINNER: (End of stress) Take
- ☐ 1. Vitamin C, 1 gram
- ☐ 2. Vitamin E, 100 I.U.
- ☐ 3. Glutamine (if needed)

OXYGENATE THRU EXERCISE: 15–20 minutes on the bike, in the pool, a run, brisk walk, dance, chop wood, lift weights or love strongly, even a trampoline.

BEDTIME: Ritually prepare for deep sleep by taking:
- ☐ 1. Calcium/magnesium, 250 mg.
- ☐ 2. 4–6 drops Passiflora (if needed)
- ☐ 3. Tryptophan (if needed)

4 DAYS TO FREEDOM **DAY #27**

WAKE-UP TIME: Take
☐ 1. Multi Vitamin/Mineral
☐ 2. Vitamin C, 1 gram
☐ 3. Vitamin E, 100 I.U.
☐ 4. Phenylalanine (if needed)
☐ 5. Gotu Kola herbal tea, 1 cup

HALF-WAY THRU: Take
(mid-morning)
☐ 1. Vitamin C, 1 gram
☐ 2. Vitamin E, 100 I.U.
☐ 3. Choline, 1 gram
☐ 4. Lecithin, 1 tablespoon

LUNCH (EAT! Even a bit) *Then* take
☐ 1. Vitamin C, 1 gram
☐ 2. Calcium/magnesium, 250 mg.

ALMOST THRU TIME: Take
☐ 1. B-Complex, 50–100 mg.
☐ 2. Vitamin C, 1 gram
☐ 3. Vitamin E, 100 I.U.
☐ 4. Phenylalanine (if needed)

DINNER: (End of stress) Take
☐ 1. Vitamin C, 1 gram
☐ 2. Vitamin E, 100 I.U.
☐ 3. Glutamine (if needed)

OXYGENATE THRU EXERCISE: 15–20 minutes on the bike, in the pool, a run, brisk walk, dance, chop wood, lift weights or love strongly, even a trampoline.

BEDTIME: Ritually prepare for deep sleep by taking:
☐ 1. Calcium/magnesium, 250 mg.
☐ 2. 4–6 drops Passiflora (if needed)
☐ 3. Tryptophan (if needed)

3 DAYS TO FREEDOM **DAY #28**

WAKE-UP TIME: Take
☐ 1. Multi Vitamin/Mineral
☐ 2. Vitamin C, 1 gram
☐ 3. Vitamin E, 100 I.U.
☐ 4. Phenylalanine (if needed)
☐ 5. Gotu Kola herbal tea, 1 cup

HALF-WAY THRU: Take
(mid-morning)
☐ 1. Vitamin C, 1 gram
☐ 2. Vitamin E, 100 I.U.
☐ 3. Choline, 1 gram
☐ 4. Lecithin, 1 tablespoon

LUNCH (EAT! Even a bit) *Then* take
☐ 1. Vitamin C, 1 gram
☐ 2. Calcium/magnesium, 250 mg.

ALMOST THRU TIME: Take
☐ 1. B-Complex, 50–100 mg.
☐ 2. Vitamin C, 1 gram
☐ 3. Vitamin E, 100 I.U.
☐ 4. Phenylalanine (if needed)

DINNER: (End of stress) Take
☐ 1. Vitamin C, 1 gram
☐ 2. Vitamin E, 100 I.U.
☐ 3. Glutamine (if needed)

OXYGENATE THRU EXERCISE: 15–20 minutes on the bike, in the pool, a run, brisk walk, dance, chop wood, lift weights or love strongly, even a trampoline.

BEDTIME: Ritually prepare for deep sleep by taking:
☐ 1. Calcium/magnesium, 250 mg.
☐ 2. 4–6 drops Passiflora (if needed)
☐ 3. Tryptophan (if needed)

2 DAYS TO FREEDOM **DAY #29**

WAKE-UP TIME: Take
☐ 1. Multi Vitamin/Mineral
☐ 2. Vitamin C, 1 gram
☐ 3. Vitamin E, 100 I.U.
☐ 4. Phenylalanine (if needed)
☐ 5. Gotu Kola herbal tea, 1 cup

HALF-WAY THRU: Take
(mid-morning)
☐ 1. Vitamin C, 1 gram
☐ 2. Vitamin E, 100 I.U.
☐ 3. Choline, 1 gram
☐ 4. Lecithin, 1 tablespoon

LUNCH (EAT! Even a bit) *Then* take
☐ 1. Vitamin C, 1 gram
☐ 2. Calcium/magnesium, 250 mg.

ALMOST THRU TIME: Take
☐ 1. B-Complex, 50–100 mg.
☐ 2. Vitamin C, 1 gram
☐ 3. Vitamin E, 100 I.U.
☐ 4. Phenylalanine (if needed)

DINNER: (End of stress) Take
☐ 1. Vitamin C, 1 gram
☐ 2. Vitamin E, 100 I.U.
☐ 3. Glutamine (if needed)

OXYGENATE THRU EXERCISE: 15–20 minutes on the bike, in the pool, a run, brisk walk, dance, chop wood, lift weights or love strongly, even a trampoline.

BEDTIME: Ritually prepare for deep sleep by taking:
☐ 1. Calcium/magnesium, 250 mg.
☐ 2. 4–6 drops Passiflora (if needed)
☐ 3. Tryptophan (if needed)

DAY OF FREEDOM **DAY #30***

FREE AT LAST!!

WAKE-UP TIME: Take

☐ 1. Multi Vitamin/Mineral
☐ 2. Vitamin C, 1 gram
☐ 3. Vitamin E, 100 I.U.
☐ 4. Phenylalanine (if needed)
☐ 5. Gotu Kola herbal tea, 1 cup

HALF-WAY THRU: Take
(mid-morning)

☐ 1. Vitamin C, 1 gram
☐ 2. Vitamin E, 100 I.U.
☐ 3. Choline, 1 gram
☐ 4. Lecithin, 1 tablespoon

LUNCH (EAT! Even a bit) *Then* take

☐ 1. Vitamin C, 1 gram
☐ 2. Calcium/magnesium, 250 mg.

ALMOST THRU TIME: Take

☐ 1. B-Complex, 50–100 mg.
☐ 2. Vitamin C, 1 gram
☐ 3. Vitamin E, 100 I.U.
☐ 4. Phenylalanine (if needed)

DINNER: (End of stress) Take

☐ 1. Vitamin C, 1 gram
☐ 2. Vitamin E, 100 I.U.
☐ 3. Glutamine (if needed)

OXYGENATE THRU EXERCISE: 15–20 minutes on the bike, in the pool, a run, brisk walk, dance, chop wood, lift weights or love strongly, even a trampoline.

**Do not drop all supplements at once. Gradually reduce your amino acids; drop the adrenal extract and see what changes occur; skip the Passiflora and see how you sleep; ALWAYS maintain your multi vitamin/mineral; vitamins C & E; B-Complex and calcium/magnesium.*

BEDTIME: Ritually prepare for deep sleep by taking:

☐ 1. Calcium/magnesium, 250 mg.
☐ 2. 4–6 drops Passiflora (if needed)
☐ 3. Tryptophan (if needed)

Chapter 3

HOW ANTIOXIDANTS HELP COCAINISTS

In the "30 Days to Freedom" plan, notice the large doses of vitamins C and E I recommend. In addition to these antioxidant nutrients your multivitamin/mineral tablet will likely contain at least 20,000 I.U. of vitamin A and 20–50 micrograms of the mineral selenium.

"ACE—Selenium", is a good way to remember these helpful nutrients. They work in many ways, but for the purposes of discussing this treatment program, in this chapter let's look at how they act to "reduce the incidence of cancer" by scavenging free radicals which can be "toxic, mutagenic and carcinogenic" (Simic and Karel, 1980).

Recall that cocaine increases the utilization of noradrenaline (norepinephrine) at the nerve endings. This substance goes on to produce a body chemical, *adrenochrome,* which can be converted into *adrenolutin,* "a toxin which causes hallucinations and bizarre sensory dysperception" (Lesser, 1980). This is one theory of schizophrenia. The eminent nutrition-oriented psychiatrist, Michael Lesser, M.D., speculates that vitamin C may act here by detoxifying the *adrenochrome* into a *non-toxic* (and nonhallucinogenic) substance called leuco-adrenochrome.

In this sequence of reactions free radical damagers are formed which will try to bond with many molecules in the body. These newly formed substances are usually toxic.

Now, our body normally controls free radicals formed during our metabolic processes, by use of enzymes. However, when we are under constant stress or use drugs such as cocaine or amphetamine-like compounds, more adrenaline is produced which makes *more* damaging free radical compounds. Our normal enzyme quenching systems are inadequate to control this increased production so we need to *add antioxidants* to our foods and take supplements to reduce or eliminate these harmful by-products.

This explanation is greatly simplified. An important text which describes how free radical reactions work to produce toxic substances and how antioxidants work to suppress these reactions is available for further study. It is titled "Autoxidation in Food and Biological Systems", edited by Michael G. Simic and Marcus Karel (1980).

One article in this book names the actual damaging free radical formed during the breakdown of adrenaline. It is a *superoxide radical* which the authors say *attacks* the *cell membrane,* making a hole in it. The cell membrane is a "prime target for peroxidative damage (from oxidized lipids)".

So, if you have been using a great deal of cocaine you have greatly increased the amount of free radical damagers in your body, and you need the antioxidants to scavenge them, rendering them harmless.

Chapter 4

LOOKING CLOSELY (At the Vitamins, Minerals, Amino Acids, Herbs, and Other Things You Will Use)

Multi Vitamin/Mineral:

This is the backbone of your nutrient therapy and should be selected with great care. Do *not* buy a discount or supermarket multi vitamin. Stick to a reputable manufacturer.

Here is how to select your brand:

(1) How much Vitamin E does it contain? This is the *most expensive* ingredient in a "multi" and often in short supply. A good formula will contain *at least* 150 I.U.

(2) *Biotin:* Make sure it contains *at least* 100 mcg. (micrograms). This is another highly expensive

nutrient and a good indicator of the general quality of your over-all formula. Essential in forming nucleic acids, glycogen, and required in the synthesis of several amino acids.

(3) *Chromium:* It should contain between 100–200 *micrograms* (mcg.) of this mineral which is of critical importance in proper functioning of glucose and carbohydrate metabolism. This trace mineral has a key role in preventing and controlling adult-onset diabetes, as part of the "glucose-tolerance-factor", or GTF (see Weiner, 1981).

(4) *Selenium:* Make sure your "multi" contains *at least* 20 mcg. of this antioxidant. The safe limit is about 400–500 mcg. daily, including food sources.

(5) Of course the "multi" you select will also contain other nutrients. I have listed those which are the keys to *evaluating a superior formula.*

Here are the nutrients generally found in a quality formula:

WHAT TO LOOK FOR IN A "MULTI" FORMULA

Nutrient	**Dosage Range**	
Vitamin A	20,000 I.U.	25,000 I.U.
Vitamin D	400 I.U.	1,000 I.U.
Vitamin E	150 I.U.	400 I.U.
Vitamin C	150 mg.	
Vitamin B-1	50 mg.	100 mg.
Vitamin B-2	50 mg.	100 mg.
Vitamin B-6	50 mg.	100 mg.
Niacinamide	50 mg.	100 mg.
Vitamin B-12	50 mcg.	100 mcg.

Nutrient	Dosage Range	
Choline	75 mg.	200 mg.
Inositol	50 mg.	100 mg.
PABA	50 mg.	100 mg.
Pantothenic Acid	50 mg.	100 mg.
Biotin	100 mcg.	300 mcg.
Folic Acid	400 mcg.	
Iodine	150 mcg.	
Calcium	50 mg.	150 mg.
Magnesium	25 mg.	75 mg.
Iron	18 mg.	30 mg.
Copper	0.5 mg.	2 mg.
Zinc	15 mg.	30 mg.
Manganese	5 mg	20 mg.
Chromium	100 mcg.	200 mcg.
Selenium	20 mcg.	40 mcg.

Be sure to take this "backbone" vitamin/mineral formula every day. Then, build upon it with the full range of supplements recommended in my 30-day treatment program, as follows:

VITAMINS

Vitamin A

Vitamin A is often associated with maintenance of proper vision and prevention of night blindness, but it does much more than that. A powerful antioxidant and free radical deactivator, this valuable vitamin helps to protect against the potential damage from free radicals released during the sped-up metabolic processes of cocaine use. It helps to stabilize the cellular membranes. It is also an important stimulant to the immune system, and protects the thymus, the gland associated with the immune system.

Because it promotes the normal development of epithelial tissue, vitamin A protects against cancer of the skin, lung, and other epithelial tissues, where nearly half of all human cancers begin. It has also been shown to lower blood cholesterol in people with high cholesterol levels.

Vitamin A is needed in the manufacture of the anti-stress hormones of the adrenal cortex, and so vitamin A is used up under stressful conditions. Signs of vitamin A deficiency include insomnia, fatigue, depression, and nerve pains in the extremities. After the stress of cocaine abuse, and during the stress of withdrawal, vitamin A is a crucial supplement.

Because it is soluble in fat rather than water, vitamin A can be toxic in excessive doses, since it can accumulate in the fatty tissues of the body. It is important, therefore, to take vitamin A with other antioxidants such as vitamins E and C and the mineral selenium, since these will help protect vitamin A from oxidation, thereby reducing the requirement for vitamin A itself.

Vitamin C

It will be of interest to the recovering cocaine addict to know that vitamin C has been used to help narcotics addicts achieve a smooth, symptom-free withdrawal from drugs such as codeine, morphine, meperidine or heroin. This therapy, which combines large doses of vitamin C with a high-protein diet, was pioneered by Drs. Irwin Stone and Alfred Libby, who report that their subjects were able to get off drugs because of the feeling of well-being produced by the vitamin C. Dr. Libby says that this treatment is equally effective in withdrawing from tobacco, alcohol, or just about any substance, provided that the abuser is motivated to quit his or her habit. Cocaine users should be heartened by this little-publicized but important clinical finding.

Vitamin C plays an important role in combating fatigue, listlessness, confusion, and depression, as well as acting as a tranquilizer for the anxious and helping insomnia. Thus, vitamin C is an important element of our program, helping to control many of the troublesome symptoms of withdrawal from cocaine.

The reason why vitamin C is so beneficial for these mental symptoms is that it plays a key role in the production of neurotransmitters in the brain, which produce a natural "high" that many seekers of bliss consider superior to anything that drugs can yield.

Vitamin C is severely depleted by stress, both mental and physical, and in our modern environment, with pollution, psychological stresses, the use of cigarettes, and exposure to other vitamin C-depleting influences—including cocaine use—it is no wonder that we require large doses of this truly "miraculous" substance.

People sometimes wonder why large doses of vitamin C should be so magically able to help against such a wide range of problems; perhaps we need to realize that as human beings we need not necessarily be susceptible to infection, slow wound healing, allergies, heart disease, cancer, and mental distress, and that by taking large doses of vitamin C we are returning to a more *normal* level of functioning.

Of interest to the cocaine abuser is vitamin C's role as an antioxidant and free radical deactivator, helping to protect against the dangerous free radicals that are released through the accelerated metabolic processes of the cocainist.

Vitamin C has also been shown to reduce serum cholesterol in some people, and to protect against atherosclerosis. It is a powerful detoxifier, helping to overcome the ill effects of heavy metals, chemicals in air pollution, carcinogenic substances, poisons, and radiation. It helps combat the undesirable side effects of many medications and may also protect against the ill effects of many of the toxic substances used to cut cocaine (see Appendix 3 for common adulterants in cocaine).

Vitamin C functions as an anti-cancer agent by combating the formation of cancer-causing nitrosamines in the bowels. It not only protects against cancer, but it is also used in high doses to treat existing cancers. It has an important role in the immune system, helping us to resist disease. It is also important in the formation of collagen, the connective tissue throughout the body, whose breakdown is partly responsible for the aging process. Collagen is also involved in wound healing, which is promoted by vitamin C. Since this vitamin helps maintain the bones, cartilage and connective tissue, it is an important adjunct to any exercise program, protecting against damage to the spine and joints from jogging and other forms of exercise.

Vitamin C has a powerful synergistic effect on the other water-soluble antioxidants, and helps vitamin E keep from being used up when it deactivates peroxide molecules.

It is easy to see why vitamin C is considered an essential dietary factor in promoting a healthy long life!

Vitamin E

One of the most notable functions of vitamin E in terms of cocaine withdrawal is its ability to facilitate the transport of oxygen to the blood. Vitamin E is a crucial part of our rehabilitation program, helping to fight fatigue and oxygen starvation in the cells to produce a nontoxic, natural high. The relationship between vitamin E and aerobic exercise is so important that it will be discussed separately in the next chapter.

Vitamin E is a very effective antioxidant and free radical deactivator, protecting the structural integrity of the cell membranes and helping neutralize the damaging effect of smog and other environmental pollutants, including the carbon monoxide in cigarette smoke. It is the only known antioxidant which protects cellular structures by preventing lipid peroxidation—the breakdown of fatty substances which releases dangerous free radicals. As we have seen, these free radicals are not only an important factor in the aging process but are also suspected to be involved as initiators of cancers (Johnson, 1983).

Vitamin E also appears to prevent the accumulation of cholesterol in the arteries and protects against the formation of abnormal blood clots which can result in heart attack or stroke.

It is reported to have a calming effect on nervous or exhausted individuals, and has helped to relieve the mental symptoms of menopause. One of its earliest discovered functions was the prevention of sterility in rats, and although its reputation as a "sex vitamin" was exaggerated, it does help protect the sex hormones as well as other substances in the body against oxidation.

Vitamin E is most effective when it is taken with other antioxidants, such as the mineral selenium, vitamin C, and the amino acid cystine. It should be taken with meals that contain some fats or oils, since it is necessary for such foods to induce bile flow in order for the vitamin E to be properly assimilated.

Vitamin B Complex

The B vitamins are grouped together because they tend to occur in the same foods and they do similar work in the body. They should be taken in combination as B complex because some of the B vitamins help the body to use others.

In general, the B vitamins are known for their ability to help deal with stress. For the minimally oxygen-starved, overstressed system of the withdrawing cocainist, they are an essential factor in dealing with depression and fatigue, maintaining energy, and calming the nerves.

One B vitamin, choline, is so important in treating the nervous systems of cocaine users that it will be dealt with separately. Other members of the vitamin B complex also serve functions which are of special help in getting off coke.

Pantothenic acid is an important anti-stress vitamin. It is also involved in the production of acetylcholine in the brain and nervous system, and in energy metabolism.

Inositol may be helpful in combating insomnia.

Its mild anti-anxiety effect often makes it a useful, *natural* alternative to mild prescription tranquilizers.

Vitamin B_1, or thiamin, is involved in the conversion of blood sugar to caloric energy in the body. During stressful periods it can give a boost to your energy level. Thiamin can be depleted by poor diet, and by overuse of caffeine and tobacco. The need for thiamin is also increased by the use of cocaine.

Niacin (vitamin B_3) helps form the active portion of co-enzymes that are essential in tissue oxidation. It can relieve the hallucinations and delusions of cocaine withdrawal, as well as correcting disturbances in mood and energy. In high doses niacin has been found effective in treating some forms of schizophrenia. Taken in combination with a high-protein diet, niacin makes it possible for some people to decrease their intake of tranquilizers.

Niacin also helps prevent many symptoms of aging. It improves the oxygen-carrying ability of the red blood cells and improves circulation; thus, it can contribute significantly to producing that natural high that the oxygen-starved cocaine addict craves.

The chemical difference between niacinamide and niacin is that niacin contains an organic acid group and niacinamide contains an amino group. Niacinamide does not produce vasodilation (flushing) as niacin does. The niacin form is found in plants while niacinamide is found in animal life.

Vitamin B_6, or pyridoxine, is a co-enzyme which facilitates the release of glycogen from the liver and glycogen phosphate from muscle. It stimulates dreaming (Pfeiffer, 1975) and protects against heart attacks (Williams, 1973).

Vitamin B_{12}, or cobalamin, is an anti-stress and

anti-fatigue vitamin which is useful in dealing with general tiredness and nervousness. It participates in methyl group metabolism in the body as a co-enzyme in the chemical conversion of methyl malonyl CoA to succinyl CoA. Succinyl CoA is involved in energy-yielding metabolic reactions. Only a few mcg. are actually absorbed through the intestinal wall, so small amounts are adequate.

Vitamin B_{15}, *pangamic acid*, is an extremely interesting substance which seems to prevent oxygen starvation in the tissues by stimulating normal oxidative metabolism.

It functions as an intermediary metabolite enhancing numerous biochemical processes through transmethylations at the cellular level. During metabolism, B_{15} gives rise to glycine, the simplest amino acid with numerous functions, and two available methyl groups. These metabolites work together to improve the quality of the body's nutritional environment, particularly under hypoxia conditions. Containing a methyl donor, this nutrient enhances oxygen utilization at the cellular level, facilitates adaptation to hypoxia conditions, and detains and diminishes lactic acid build up in the blood. As a result, *fatigue is postponed and endurance is increased.*

Russian researchers report it has many uses, including the treatment of alcoholism and other drug addictions. Unfortunately, in the United States federal and state authorities are suspicious of this vitamin and it is not presently available.

All in all, the B complex can be very helpful in dealing with the depression, fatigue, and weakness that are so often part of withdrawal of cocaine.

Choline and Lecithin

Choline is generally considered one of the B vitamins, even though it can be manufactured in the body from other nutrients. It is a precursor of lecithin, a "super food" commonly derived from soy oil.

Lecithin and choline are of particular interest for someone withdrawing from cocaine because of their effect on the nervous system. The body manufactures acetylcholine from choline and lecithin in the diet. Acetylcholine is the neurotransmitter responsible for the transmission of messages from one nerve cell to another in the brain; it regulates the activity of muscles and of the parasympathetic nervous system. It is required for memory, appetite, and sexual behavior, and regulates our responsiveness to internal and external stimuli. It controls our ability to "turn off" the outside environment so we can sleep.

Physical restlessness that prevents sleep, often a problem for the cocainist or ex-user, may respond to stimulation of acetylcholine production; this can be accomplished by taking choline and lecithin supplements.

A deficiency of acetylcholine can also lead to depression, and hence choline and lecithin can have an anti-depressant effect as well as an anxiety-relieving effect for people getting off cocaine. Because of its calmative effect, lecithin is sometimes used in place of minor tranquilizers.

Lecithin has the important additional benefit of helping to dissolve cholesterol accumulations, thus protecting the cardiovascular system as well as the nervous system.

In order for lecithin and choline to be converted to acetylcholine in the body, there must be adequate pantothenic acid (a B vitamin) present. Thus it is important to take a vitamin B complex supplement along with these important nutrients in order for them to help combat anxiety and depression.

THE MINERALS

Calcium/Magnesium

One of the troublesome symptoms of cocaine withdrawal is muscle cramping and twitching. These symptoms are helped by the minerals calcium and magnesium, which act as natural tranquilizers and muscle relaxants.

Calcium is the most plentiful mineral element in the body. Most of it goes to make up our bones and teeth, while a very small proportion in the soft tissues and blood has a crucial effect on nerve function. Extreme calcium deficiency can produce twitching of the muscles, cramps, irritation, confusion, even convulsions; while lesser degrees of deficiency can result in depression, irritability, impaired memory, and calf cramps.

Magnesium acts as a natural tranquilizer for the nervous system, and has been used to treat anxiety, depression, insomnia, and hyperactivity in children. It is also essential for normal heart function. It regulates the critical balances of various substances in the body, such as sodium and chloride, calcium and phosphorus.

Calcium and magnesium should be taken in the ratio of 2:1. If there is too much or too little magnesium in relation to calcium, the body won't be able to absorb enough calcium.

Selenium

Selenium, the other mineral element in our treatment program, can be highly poisonous in too-high doses. Because the toxic dose is very close to the dose for dietary supplementation, nutritionists have been very cautious in recommending selenium as a supplement. However, we now know that it is an extremely important trace mineral, acting as an antioxidant like vitamin E, and a free radical deactivator. It slows down aging, prevents heart and blood vessel disease, and may help to prevent cancer (Shamberger, 1969).

As with the other antioxidants in our withdrawal plan, selenium helps to protect against damage from free radicals released by the sped-up metabolism of the cocainist.

Adequate selenium is required in order for vitamin E to perform many of its functions. It enhances the efficiency of vitamin E, while at the same time vitamin E increases the body's tolerance to the potentially toxic selenium. Besides their antioxidant and anti-free radical activity, vitamin E and selenium together also improve the functioning of the immune system, boosting resistance to disease.

THE AMINO ACIDS

The three amino acids 1-glutamine, 1-phenylalanine, and 1-tyrosine all stimulate nerve and brain functioning, providing the boost that the cocainist has been seeking through the use of the drug.

1-Glutamine*

Glutamic acid, one of the "non-essential" amino acids, has a unique function in brain metabolism. It is the only substance other than glucose which can serve as a fuel for the brain, and so it has been shown to give a lift from fatigue and improve intelligence, among other benefits. Glutamic acid also protects the body by serving as a buffer against excess ammonia, in what is known as the "citric acid cycle".

Although glutamic acid provides energy for the brain, it isn't possible for the brain to derive glutamic acid directly from food, owing to the protective blood-brain barrier which allows only a very few chemicals to enter the brain directly from the blood. However it *is* possible to increase the glutamic acid in the brain by providing the proper building blocks in the diet. This is why 1-glutamine is recommended as a dietary supplement. This form of glutamic acid can readily cross the blood barrier into the brain, where it is quickly converted into glutamic acid.

Besides its function as a source of energy for the brain, 1-glutamine has also been shown to protect against the poisonous effects of alcohol and to stop a craving for alcohol. Studies have shown that 1-glutamine helps to fight fatigue, depression, and impotence, and it has been used successfully against schizophrenia, senility and mental retardation.

Thus, 1-glutamine as a dietary supplement is a

**In this chapter and throughout the book, we use the "1-" designation interchangeably with the more general name for an amino acid (such as 1-cystine, the same as cystine). We do this for the sake of simplicity.*

natural source of energy and alertness that the cocaine addict craves. (Rogers, 1955; Shive, 1957; Williams, 1973.)

1-Phenylalanine

The amino acid phenylalanine creates a natural sense of well-being, owing to its role in producing the neurotransmitters adrenaline and noradrenaline, as well as other important hormones. This nutrient appears to help overcome depression, increase mental alertness, improve memory, control allergies, and aid weight loss by suppressing appetite.

The body's requirement for 1-phenylalanine is higher than for the other amino acids. It is the raw material that produces several compounds known as catecholamines—neurotransmitters which include adrenaline and noradrenaline. The adrenal medulla and the nerve cells can only manufacture these catecholamines when there is enough phenylalanine (or its derivative, tyrosine) in the blood. Adrenaline and noradrenaline are responsible for a positive, elevated mood of alertness—the "natural high" which the cocainist tries to mimic through the use of drugs.

Medical researchers, as well as drug abusers, have often tried to produce this state of alertness through the use of drugs such as amphetamines, which cause the release of noradrenaline and block its return to storage. However, such an artificial manipulation ultimately leads to an aggravation of the original problem as the neurotransmitter is depleted. It is a much more natural solution to provide adequate levels of dietary 1-phenylalanine, thereby assuring that normal levels of noradrenaline will be maintained in the brain and nerves, providing a boost in energy and alertness that is not followed by a "crash".

In addition to making this stimulating amino acid a major component of the 30-day program, in the form of capsules, foods rich in it are named in Chapter 6, "Protein Meals for Repair". (Stein, 1975; Goldberg, 1980; Gelenberg, 1980.)

1-Tyrosine

Tyrosine is another amino acid which helps to overcome depression, increase mental alertness, and improve memory. Like phenylalanine, tyrosine is involved in the manufacture of the neurotransmitters adrenaline and noradrenaline, which are responsible for an elevated, positive mood.

If there is sufficient 1-phenylalanine in the body, the liver can manufacture adequate tyrosine from the phenylalanine. Otherwise, 1-tyrosine can be taken as a separate supplement.

In one study, 1-tyrosine supplementation was shown to control anxiety and long-standing depression; patients who had previously been treated for these problems with amphetamines were able to discontinue or reduce their dosage of the drugs.

Allergy sufferers and those on weight loss programs have also had positive responses to 1-tyrosine, which is a much preferred way to control appetite as opposed to the use of amphetamines, P.P.A. or other "diet pills". (Gelenberg, 1980; Goldberg, 1980; Growden, 1979.)

L-Tryptophan *(A natural sedative)*

Unlike the "psychic energizers" glutamine, phenylalanine, and tyrosine, the amino acid tryptophan has a calming effect on the nervous system. Tryptophan is well known for its ability to alleviate insomnia. It reduces anxiety, depression and pain as well as improving sleep.

L-tryptophan works as a building block for the neurotransmitter serotonin. Unlike drugs used to treat insomnia and anxiety, tryptophan does not suppress central nervous system functioning, but rather restores normal function by being available for the body to use in making serotonin as needed.

Tryptophan has other important functions as well. Recently it has been discovered that heart attacks are often triggered by irregular heartbeats or arterial spasms due to a lack of serotonin. For this reason, L-tryptophan supplementation can conceivably reduce the risk of this type of heart attack, which accounts for more than 15 percent of heart disease deaths, by making the heart less susceptible to stress-induced changes.

Although tryptophan occurs naturally in many high-protein foods, its concentration is usually small compared to that of other amino acids. For this reason it is wise to take it as a supplement so it is not diluted by the other amino acids.

Some L-tryptophan is used to make the B vitamin niacin, in people who are deficient in this vitamin. Therefore you should maintain an adequate intake of niacin if you want to get the full benefit of the tryptophan; this is accomplished by taking the B complex and multivitamin supplements recommended. (Passwater, Newsletter.)

L-Cystine *(An anti-toxicant)*

L-cystine is the stable form of the sulfur-containing amino acid cystine. This amino acid serves an important protective function for cocaine users. It contains the sulfhydryl group (an atom of sulfur and an atom of hydrogen) which is a component of the important metabolite Coenzyme A, which participates in a great many vital reactions in the body.

L-cystine helps to destroy harmful chemicals in the body such as acetaldehyde and free radicals produced by smoking, drinking, and accelerated metabolic processes. Thus it works with the vitamin and mineral antioxidants and free radical scavengers to protect against damage from free radical action, which might otherwise be increased through cocaine use. It also helps to prevent brain and liver damage from alcohol, and protects against radiation, heavy metals, and other harmful substances in the body.

It appears also that L-cystine is necessary for the proper utilization of vitamin B_6. A number of chronic degenerative diseases, both mental and physical, seem to be caused by a disorder in the utilization of B_6; hence the real, underlying cause may be an L-cystine deficiency. (Colombetti, 1971; Philpott, 1979.)

ADRENAL EXTRACT

The adrenal glands, located on top of the kidneys, consist of two parts: an inner core, or medulla, and the outer shell, or cortex. It's in the medulla that we produce adrenaline, the survival hormone that boosts mental and physical functioning to deal with sudden stress. The adrenal medulla also produces noradrenaline, which is the nervous system's version of adrenaline and functions somewhat similarly. In the adrenal cortex, other hormones are produced—those which regulate the stress response, those that control mineral balance, and some sex hormones.

As we have seen, cocaine works between the nerve endings to mimic the "rush" of adrenalin. It also stimulates the adrenal gland itself, as do many other factors, including alcohol, tobacco, caffeine, drugs, refined sugars and starches, overwork, infections or lack of rest. When the adrenal glands are overstimulated, we enter into a state of adrenal exhaustion. This condition is marked by low blood sugar, fatigue, lethargy, depression, irritability, inability to concentrate, weakness, and poor appetite. It is no accident that these symptoms sound very much like the "crash" that follows the cocaine high!

Taking adrenal extract tablets helps to stimulate adrenal function when the glands are in this sluggish, exhausted state. Adrenal stimulation also depletes vitamin C, which is highly concentrated in the gland. This is why vitamin C is such an important component of our 30-day program.

HERBS YOU WILL NEED*

Passionflower or Passiflora *(Passiflora incarnata)*

As a sedative, Passionflower has qualities unlike those of any other herb. It is very effective, with a

**These write-ups are quoted from WEINER'S HERBAL, published by Stein & Day, 1980.*

pleasant taste, and yet surprisingly gentle. It is helpful in a variety of ailments, from insomnia, dysmenorrhea, nervous tension, and fatigue, to muscle spasms. It can be used with safety even for small children.

Passiflora incarnata may be our best tranquilizer yet. The dried leaves and stems both induce a natural sleep and calm hyperactive people.

This plant drug is used in Italy to treat hyperactive children; and in the Yucatan it is an old remedy for insomnia, hysteria, and convulsions in children. Interestingly, the early Algonquin Indians brewed this woody vine to soothe their nerves. The state flower of Tennessee appears to be a useful bridge between traditional medicine and modern ills, especially anxiety states. Physicians could well recommend this plant to patients who want to wean themselves from synthetic sleeping pills and tranquilizers.

Surprisingly, one kind of Passionflower *(P. quadrangularis,* or Giant Granadilla) was recently found to contain serotonin. Low levels of this compound in the cerebrospinal fluid of patients with chronic depression have led some researchers to speculate that adding it to circulating blood would relieve states of depression. This may be confirmed by the fact that LSD-like compounds which are used to induce clinical psychoses are known to have potent anti-serotonin activity; perhaps Passionflower therefore acts as a natural calming agent by promoting the transmission of subtle nerve impulses. It appears to aid concentration, alter perception, and gently shift mood.

Utilized since its "discovery" by early Jesuit missionaries in South America, Passionflower has no known toxicity in small doses.

Dose: For medicinal use, ½ to 1 teaspoon of the dried herb is used to 1 cup of boiling water. The resultant infusion may be taken every 3 to 4 hours.

As a fluid-extract, 3–4 drops every 4 hours.

GOTU KOLA *(Centella asiatica)*

Gotu Kola is used primarily as a sedative, diuretic, tonic, and to accelerate healing of wounds. It is claimed to strengthen and energize the brain. In large doses it is said to act as a narcotic, causing stupor, headache, and sometimes coma.

It has been employed to alleviate bowel complaints and to treat syphilis and tubercular inflammation of the cervical lymph nodes. Its ability to aid in these and urinary tract disorders has been attributed to its demulcent properties.

Recent pharmacological studies have shown that extracts of Gotu Kola exhibit a sedative activity similar to that of *meprobamate* and *chlorpromazine!* The mode of action appears to be mainly in the cholinergic mechanism in the central nervous system.

The major active principle in this plant is most probably the triterpene glycoside asiaticoside. Asiaticoside is well tolerated when given by mouth to mice and rabbits at a single dose of 1.0 gram. This would imply that it is a relatively safe substance. When asiaticoside is implanted under the skin, or injected subcutaneously in mice, rats, guinea pigs, or rabbits, improved blood supply of connective tissue occurs. A rapid thickening of the skin is also noted in the treated animals, as well as an accelerated growth of hair and nails.

There is some evidence in humans, because of the sum total of these effects, that asiaticoside, and hence extracts of *Centella asiatica*, are useful to accelerate healing of wounds and some infectious diseases such as tuberculosis and leprosy. The microbes that cause both of these diseases are well-known to have a waxy coating that most other disease-producing organisms lack. This waxy coating prevents the body's own defense mechanisms from killing the organisms, hence it is difficult to cure both of these diseases. It is thought that asiaticoside acts to dissolve the waxy covering on the organisms, which then allows the normal defense mechanisms of the body to destroy the causative organisms of leprosy and/or tuberculosis.

It has also been shown that asiaticoside-pretreated rats (12.5 mg/kg/day/3 days, subcutaneously) who were then subjected to cold conditions, did not develop gastric ulcers. Control animals in the experiment did develop gastric ulcers under these conditions.

Gotu Kola awaits discovery and possible wide adoption by the medical establishment. Fijian healers have long known of the values of this plant; it is the most frequently utilized medicinal plant in their pharmacopoeia. It has long been known in India, and its use was probably brought to Fiji by Indian settlers.

Dose: Small doses of ½ teaspoon of the dried herb per cup of boiling water are recommended. The dose is sometimes increased, as needed, for sedative purposes.

WHY USE "SUDAFED"?

Isn't this just another drug?

Yes. With a difference! This mild drug is a synthesized version of a natural plant product which has been used as a healing tea in China for thousands of years. The plant is known as *ma huang,* grows in deserts, and had been very popular for treating asthma and other bronchial complaints.

Scientists from the University of California investigated this plant in the 1920's and discovered that it was named *Ephedra vulgaris.* They then isolated the active principle, an alkaloid named *ephedrine,* and realized that it had been known to science for about 80 years, and was used for treating asthma.

They next wanted a way to make ephedrine in the laboratory, to avoid having to collect the plant. After several trials they produced their best compound which was d,1-phenyliso-propylamine, or *amphetamine!* After a few changes to the new molecule the chemists came up with yet another substitute for this desert plant and called it *dexedrine!* Tried on people, scientists found the drugs improved mental and physical performance, particularly in people who were bored or fatigued; it seemed to suppress appetite; and, of course, it greatly increased wakefulness and alertness. Refer back to Chapter 1, Figure 1 and note the structures of cocaine, ephedrine and amphetamine. Cocaine and the other two compounds are quite dissimilar yet have "remarkably similar pharmacological properties" (Patrick, in Barchas, et al., 1977).

"SUDAFED" promotes most of the effects of sympathetic nervous system stimulants such as epinephrine (adrenaline). It stimulates the central nervous system *without raising blood sugar.* In addition, it is effective when taken orally (unlike epinephrine) and produces mild stimulation which *lasts a few hours* instead of a few minutes.

Caution!!! This over-the-counter drug is very useful during the first few days of withdrawal from cocaine or amphetamine. However, there are specific precautions so be sure to *read the package carefully.* Under no circumstances should this drug be taken for more than three days. For further information *discuss this with your physician.*

Chapter 5

OXYGEN, EXERCISE AND THE BENEFITS OF VITAMIN E

The nutrients and herbs recommended in this program need to get *to* your cells, where they act. Toxic wastes and the breakdown products of sustained cocaine or amphetamine use must be transported *out* of the body.

This is where daily exercise can play a major role in helping you "get off".

Now, many people will just not feel well enough to undertake vigorous public exercise. For them I suggest an indoor bicycle or small trampoline. By getting the blood moving rapidly you will accomplish both goals, faster. Namely to bring oxygen and the healing nutrients *in* and the toxic wastes *out*.

As the days go by and you begin to feel better try to increase your exercise to about 15 minutes each day. When you are ready to face the world again, outdoor running or brisk walking are ever popular "oxygenating" activities, easy to take up.

Now let's see why vitamin E is so heartily recommended in your 30-day program.

The Vitamin That Likes Oxygen

Aerobic capacity, otherwise known as efficiency of oxygen consumption, must be high enough to prevent muscle fatigue in any physical activity. Fatigue is a result of oxygen starvation in the blood. Numerous studies have proven that vitamin E levels decline as oxygen requirements increase, and are related to fatigue. Vitamin E, combined with aerobic exercise, increases the oxygen-carrying capacity of hemoglobin in the blood, leading to greater dynamic capabilities of the lungs. Since stores of this vitamin are depleted during stress, a case can be made for the need of vitamin E supplements to ensure physical stamina.

Discovery of vitamin E. Vitamin E was first discovered in 1922 by Dr. Herbert Evans and Dr. Kathryn Bishop of the University of California at Berkeley, and labeled "factor X" after it was recognized that this dietary constituent was essential for successful reproduction in animals. By 1925, vitamin E was adopted into the vitamin family, following the system of alphabetic designation of its predecessors.

Sterility was the first condition noted in vitamin E deficiency. Research over the next ten years revealed numerous deficiency states, the most noteworthy being nutritional muscular dystrophy in mammals. In 1936, Dr. Evans first isolated vitamin

E from wheat germ oil, which has the highest concentration of the vitamin among all plant foods.

Other rich natural sources of vitamin E are salad oils, fats, seeds (especially almonds and peanuts), and margarine. Some green leafy vegetables contain significant amounts of E, as do fresh asparagus and mangoes. However, processed, packaged, and stored foods may be notoriously deficient in vitamin E activity; 80 percent or more of vitamin E is lost in converting whole wheat to white bread, with freezing of vegetables also causing great losses.

Vitamin E occurs as four different compounds called tocopherols. The name "tocopherol" is derived from the Greek *tokos* (offspring) and *pherein* (to bear). It is no wonder that shortly after its discovery, vitamin E became commonly known as the "antisterility factor". Since then, researchers throughout the world have discovered a demonstrated need of vitamin E for proper maintenance and function of skeletal muscle and cardiovascular tone.

Oxygen against cocaine. Recently, much attention has been focused on the influence of vitamin E on muscular activity. Numerous claims have been cited on the value of vitamin E in postponing fatigue. In an address to the Japanese Society for Sports Medicine, Dr. Jyunichiki told a group of physicians that vitamin E facilitates the utilization of oxygen by athletes and reduces the accumulation of lactic acid, a toxic metabolite that causes muscle fatigue. By supplementing their diet with vitamin E, runners and other endurance athletes can extend their collapse point.

While runners race over the marathon course, the blood coursing through their veins often affects the results. Oxygen transport and utilization are two of the most important factors leading to success in a marathon. In competition, good marathon runners are highly efficient and use only 56 to 60 milliliters of oxygen per kilogram per minute while maintaining a pace of ten to twelve miles per hour. Trained long distance runners use up a significantly smaller proportion of their maximum capacity to consume oxygen, thus reducing negative stress and the resulting exhaustion.

When more oxygen is available in the bloodstream, stress on the heart to pump blood through the vessels is reduced. Some researchers believe that vitamin E helps promote aerobic pathways, which ensure an adequate supply of oxygen and the ability of the working cells to utilize that oxygen. Proper oxygenation of cerebral blood flow is necessary for mental as well as physical stamina, especially during this treatment program.

Although vitamin E is fat soluble, it is nontoxic, even in extremely high doses. The highest concentrations are found in the pituitary, the master gland of the body, and in the adrenals, which produce the energy-generating hormone, adrenaline. Vitamin E, in addition to iron, folic acid, B_6, B_{12}, C, copper, and protein, is a necessary component in the intricate pathways that ensure the proper function of bone marrow.

How to tell if you are deficient. The most visible sign of vitamin E deficiency is muscular dystrophy. This pernicious nutritional deficiency is comparable to scurvy, the result of vitamin C deficiency, and beriberi, the deficiency state of vitamin B_1. Early signs of vitamin E deficiency include emaciation, skin ulcers, and tremors. Cystic fibrosis, a disease that diminishes the elasticity of the lungs, is also associated with vitamin E deficiency. Muscle degeneration is the most damaging example of vitamin E deficiency.

Only recently have nutritional scientists begun to explore and understand the full significance of vitamin E's function as an antioxidant that protects the structural integrity of the cell membrane. Antioxidant is a biochemical term for any substance that prevents deterioration of cellular materials through the oxidative process, such as protecting food fats from turning rancid. As an antioxidant, vitamin E also guards against the stresses in a vigorous withdrawal program. If you choose to exercise heavily during this program, megadoses of vitamin E (1000 international units [I.U.] a day) may be valuable in reducing night leg cramps.

Protective nutrients. Among the most significant benefits of vitamin E is its ability to neutralize the formation of nitrosamines from nitrates, and to protect against the cancer-causing effects of lead, mercury, and cadmium. Vitamin E also guards against forms of toxic free radicals, substances that accelerate the aging process. Research scientists at the Linus Pauling Institute of Science and Medicine have demonstrated the role of the antioxidants vitamin C, vitamin E, and selenium in preventing the proliferation of certain cancer cells.

Recent research has emphasized the synergistic actions and the recycling of vitamin E at the expense of vitamin C. *The more vitamin C you take, the less vitamin E you need.* Here is another example of the vital role vitamin C plays in the optimal utilization of vitamin E. Vitamin C metabolism is interrelated with the mineral magnesium, to the point where the vitamin is useless without it. Neuromuscular irritability is lessened, proper elimination is promoted, body temperature regulation is influenced, and teeth are strengthened, all by the silvery white metal, magnesium.

We recommend approximately 270 mg. of magnesium daily, and more if vitamin C is supplemented in the diet, as it should be. The best sources of magnesium are wheat bran, wheat germ, soybeans, brewer's yeast, black walnuts, and roasted peanuts. Other foods rich in this important mineral are: brussels sprouts, chard, corn, peas, prunes, raisins, and spinach.

Another promising finding is the therapeutic use of vitamin E in preventing clotting disorders in women using oral contraceptives. As far as men are concerned, vitamin E may enhance the possibility of overcoming infertility and is commonly prescribed to increase sperm count and sperm activity.

Reduction in serum cholesterol is also associated with this vitamin. Recently, research enzymologists discovered that a complex relationship exists between vitamin E and the nutritional stress imposed by the presence of fats in a person's diet, especially polyunsaturated fat. People eating large amounts of vegetable oils, especially those rich in linoleic acid (e.g., corn, cottonseed, soybean), need *more* vitamin E. This is why we recommend unrefined, cold-pressed olive oil. Here is a monosaturated oil (a mix between saturated and polyunsaturated fats) with a great history among Mediterranean people known for their resistance to the diseases of aging.

Another purported benefit of vitamin E is that it improves circulation by keeping the blood density down. When the hematocrit, or red blood cell concentration, is too high, lethargic circulation can result, leading to body cells starved of their nutrients and cellular waste materials improperly eliminated. Such degenerative problems as strokes, high blood pressure, and kidney malfunctions can result.

When the fatty acids in the bloodstream oxidize or go rancid, oxygen is lost in the process. By blocking the oxidation of fatty acids, vitamin E releases more oxygen to service the body's tissues and muscles.

Medical anthropologists have reported immunity to atherosclerosis among the Masai warriors of East Africa, who herd cattle on foot, and also among the Tarahumara Indians of Mexico who take part in ceremonial runs. The diets of both groups consist mainly of unrefined vegetable grains high in vitamin E.

In 1972, reports from Swedish researchers indicated that men recovering from heart attacks, who were taking vitamin E supplements as part of their daily diet, had developed prolonged blood-clotting time. The doctors suggested that this positive change might be due to the fact that large daily doses of vitamin E depress the vitamin K-dependent coagulation factor. With a prolonged blood-clotting time, a person's blood flows more freely, helping to prevent a recurrence of heart attacks. Traditionally, doctors use such strong drugs as heparin and dicumarol to produce this effect. However, these drugs often have powerful, negative side effects not present when vitamin E is taken instead.

The combination of regular, moderate exercise and vitamin supplementation with a rational diet offers the greatest protection against the development of heart disease.

"E" against stress. In urban environments where

smog diminishes air quality, there is an increased need for antioxidants such as vitamin C, vitamin E, and selenium. Smog is an environmental stress on the oxygen-carrying potential of the circulatory system. At times, veteran runners collapse before completing marathons in urban areas. Numerous reports have cited the protective effect of vitamin E on the sensitivity of lung tissue to air pollution. The predominant oxidant in the atmosphere is smog. Vitamin E, as an antioxidant, helps to neutralize smog's damaging effects.

Hard exercise stresses the cardiovascular, respiratory, and neuromuscular systems. In long-distance running, the neuro-muscular system, especially the nerves and long muscles of the legs, experiences the greatest stress. Stress is also implicated in decreased longevity. In recent years, vitamin E has been labeled the "anti-stress factor," *because it facilitates oxygen transport to the blood.*

Cautions! Dr. William Cathcart III, an orthopedic surgeon who has worked in sports medicine and has been involved in research with Linus Pauling, cautions:

> People who take vitamin E, especially heart patients and diabetics, should do so only under proper medical advice. Because vitamin E is a strong heart stimulant, high doses can increase the blood pressure of people suffering from atherosclerosis or hypertension. Diabetics on high dosages of insulin should only take vitamin E in graduated amounts.

As a precaution, anyone considering therapeutic doses of vitamin E should consult a nutritionist or a doctor trained in nutrition.

Chapter 6

HIGH ENERGY NERVE FOODS

During your 30-day withdrawal program, you can help to maintain a high energy level by eating high-protein foods rich in the noradrenaline-pumping amino acid, phenylalanine.

The following tables list the phenylalanine and calorie content in many common foods. It isn't the purpose of these food lists to put you on a diet; you will be under enough stress simply trying to withdraw. We list the calorie content of these foods simply so that you can see how densely packed they are with phenylalanine, on a per-calorie basis.

By selecting some of the foods from each food group, and including them in your meals each day, you will help keep your energy level and spirits high. While I don't want to burden you with food restrictions, I do recommend that you avoid high-carbohydrate meals during your withdrawal program, because a diet high in starches and sugars will tend to slow you down and make you drowsy.

You may have been craving certain of the foods

on the following list—perhaps fish, or certain cheeses. The reason could well be that you needed the nerve-energy boost of their high phenylalanine content.

Some foods, such as sweets, and even fruits, have very little phenylalanine. Most vegetables are also low in phenylalanine, but there are some, such as broccoli, brussels sprouts, and other highly nourishing foods, which are quite high in phenylalanine for their calorie content. You will note that dried beans, split peas, lentils, and similar dried legumes are also high-protein energy boosters.

These lists are not meant to be exhaustive, but are only a guide to *some* of the phenylalanine-rich foods you can easily obtain for your daily meals—whether you eat at home, or in a restaurant.

Look over the following lists and see how many of your favorite foods are included. Don't hesitate to splurge on your diet during your 30-day program. When you consider how much money you will be saving by not using cocaine, you'll see you can easily afford your most craved high-ticket food items.

Caution: Remember, I am not suggesting that you *limit* your foods to those listed, but simply that they be included with *other foods* that you like each day.

How the Right Amino Acids Work to Get You "High"*

In Chapters 1 and 4, I discussed the amino acid phenylalanine, with particular emphasis on how it

**See Figure 2*

works between nerves. Recall that it is converted in the body into norepinephrine and later epinephrine, also called *adrenaline.*

The effects of adrenaline, particularly its stimulant properties, are likely increased by cocaine because cocaine blocks the recycling of natural chemical transmitters (such as norepinephrine). Acting in the *synaptic cleft* (between the axon of one nerve cell and the dendrites of the next) cocaine effectively keeps nerve transmitters such as adrenaline present, creating the same effect as if *more* nerve transmitter molecules (i.e., more adrenaline) were being released.

Remember this: adrenaline is made within the body from the amino acid phenylalanine. So, to increase our supply of this nerve transmitter *without* using cocaine I recommend that high protein *foods,* those especially *rich* in *phenylalanine,* be taken.

By the way, for those readers who may be asking "what effect does this amino acid have, if any, on oxygen flow to the brain," I quote a leading expert in the field of pharmacology: "In man, intravenous infusion of pressor doses (of adrenaline), increases both cerebral blood flow and cerebral oxygen consumption . . ." (See Goodman & Gilman.) So, if we take enough phenylalanine, through foods and via capsules, we probably achieve the same *oxygenating effect.*

HOW ADRENALINE IS MADE NATURALLY IN YOUR BODY FROM COMMON AMINO ACIDS (FOUND IN PROTEIN FOODS) (FIGURE 2)

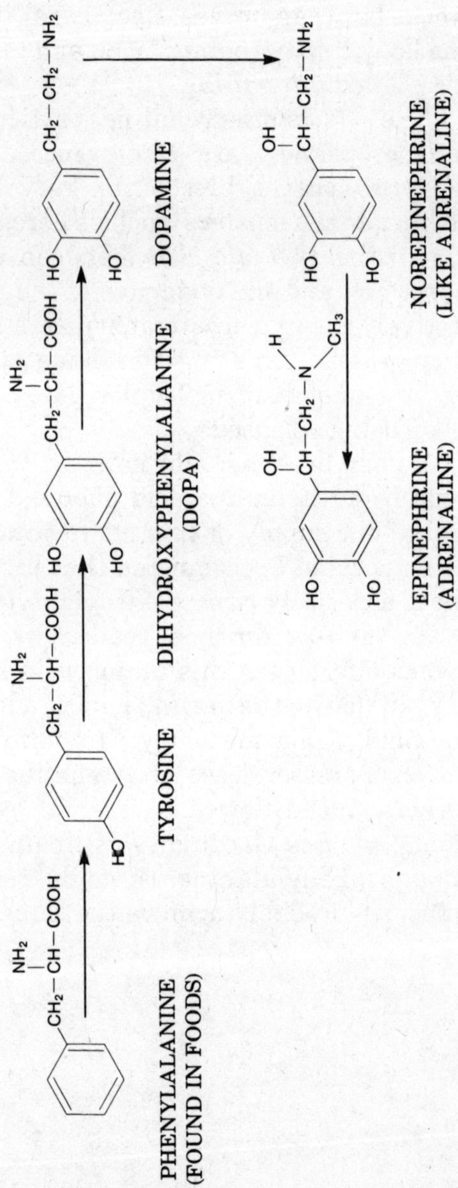

HIGH ENERGY NERVE FOODS*

Breads, Cereals and Grains	Serving size	Weight (grams)	Calories (Kcal)	Phenylalanine (mg.)
Breads				
Corn Bread, Southern Style, with Enriched Yellow Cornmeal	1 piece	45	100	152
Rye Bread, Pumpernickel	1 slice	32	79	136
Whole Wheat Bread	1 slice	23	56	117
Whole Wheat Muffins	1 average	40	103	209
Noodles, Egg, Cooked	1 cup	160	200	317
Pancakes, Homemade	1 average	45	104	173
Cereals, Ready to Eat				
Life, Quaker	1 cup	42	159	119
100% Natural, Quaker	1 oz.	28	137	152
Shredded Wheat	1 biscuit	25	89	120
Wheat Flakes	1 cup	30	114	143
Grains and Cereals, Hot				
Corn Hominy, Grits Enriched, Cooked	1 cup	242	123	131
Oatmeal/Rolled Oats, Cooked	1 cup	236	148	275
Popcorn, Popped with Fat and Salt	1½ cup	21	81	210

**Source: Bowes and Church, 1980*

Breads, Cereals and Grains	Serving size	Weight (grams)	Calories (Kcal)	Phenylalanine (mg.)
Rice, Brown, Cooked	1 cup	150	178	190
Cream of Rice, Enriched, Long Grain, Instant, Cooked	1 cup	148	161	165
Farina, Enriched, Reg., Dry	1 cup when cooked	38	140	198
Wheat Germ, Toasted	1 Tbsp.	10	39	91
Milk				
Milk, Skim	1 cup	246	89	418
Milk, Whole	1 cup	244	150	393
Yogurt, Whole	1 cup	227	141	429
Soybean Milk	1 cup	263	87	513
Cheese				
Cheddar, American	1 oz.	28	112	378
Cottage, Uncreamed (2% fat)	1 cup	226	203	1675
Cottage, Creamed	3½ oz.	100	106	704
Edam	1 oz.	28	87	416
Gouda	1 oz.	28	100	401
Gruyere	1 oz.	28	115	429
Monterey Jack	1 oz.	28	105	361
Mozzarella, Part Skim	1 oz.	28	72	359
Muenster	1 oz.	28	104	352
Parmesan, Hard	1 oz.	28	111	545
Port du Salut	1 oz.	28	99	370
Provolone	1 oz.	28	98	360
Ricotta	½ cup	124	216	689

Cheese	Serving size	Weight (grams)	Calories (Kcal)	Phenylal-anine (mg.)
Swiss, American	1 oz.	28	106	485
Tilsit	1 oz.	28	95	380
Eggs				
Boiled	1 med.	48	78	360
Fried (with 1 tsp. margarine)	1 med.	50	108	360
Omelet, Spanish	2 eggs, 4 T sauce	152	329	829
Scrambled, with milk and fat	1 med.	65	112	413
Duck Egg	1 med.	74	142	622
Fish				
Albacore, Raw	3½ oz.	100	177	936
Bass, Striped, Broiled	3½ oz.	100	228	853
Bluefish, Baked Filet	1 serving	125	199	1214
Caviar, Canned, Pressed	1 round tsp.	10	32	150
Caviar, Sturgeon, Granular	1 round tsp.	10	26	119
Cod, Broiled	4 oz. before cooking	95	162	960
Crab, Steamed	3½ oz.	100	93	830
Flounder or Sole, Baked	1 serving	100	202	1110
Halibut, Broiled	1 serving	125	214	1166
Lobster, Boiled or Broiled (edible portion 36%)	1¾ lb.	334	308	940
Mackerel, Broiled Filet	1 filet	130	300	1047
Pompano, Broiled	3½ oz.	100	284	849

Fish	Serving size	Weight (grams)	Calories (Kcal)	Phenylal-anine (mg.)
Salmon, Broiled or Baked	1 small serving	100	182	999
Sardines, Atlantic, Canned in Oil	8 medium	100	311	762
Snapper, Red or Gray, Raw	3½ oz.	100	93	733
Meats				
Beef				
Arm/Blade, Lean Only	2 slices	41	90	593
Club Steak, Lean Only	1 steak	55	108	658
Corned, Medium Fat, Canned	3 slices	85	184	884
Cubed Steak	3½ oz.	100	261	1336
Flank Steak, Lean Only	1 serving	75	158	1057
Hamburger, Lean	1 patty	86	140	1066
Porterhouse Steak, Lean Only	1 steak	54	102	605
Rib Roast, Lean Only	2 slices	41	70	453
Rib Steak, Lean Only	1 serving	43	73	506
Round, Bottom, Lean Only, Broiled	1 slice	86	205	1255
Rump, Lean Only, Pot Roasted	2 slices	37	77	494
Sirloin, Lean Only, Broiled	1 slice	77	128	856
Sirloin Tip, Lean Only, Roasted	1 slice	44	74	551

Beef	Serving size	Weight (grams)	Calories (Kcal)	Phenylal-anine (mg.)
T-Bone, Lean Only, Broiled	1 steak	59	116	642
Tenderloin, Lean Only, Broiled	1 steak	52	107	625
Chicken				
Broiler, Raw	3½ oz.	100	151	811
Fryer, Breast, Raw	3½ oz.	100	104	937
Fryer, Drum-stick, Raw	3½ oz.	100	112	824
Game				
Duck, Domestic, Flesh Only, Raw	3½ oz.	100	165	842
Rabbit, Domes-tic, Flesh Only, Raw	3½ oz.	100	162	793
Lamb				
Arm Chop, Lean Only	2 chops	59	110	671
Leg, Lean Only, Roasted	2 slices	61	107	715
Loin Chop, Lean Only	2 chops	70	130	797
Organ Meats				
Beef Heart, Lean, Braised	3½ oz.	100	179	874
Beef Kidneys, Braised	3½ oz.	100	252	911
Beef Liver, Raw	3½ oz.	100	135	993
Calf Liver, Raw	3½ oz.	100	140	958
Calf Liver, Fried	3½ oz.	100	261	1133
Chicken Liver, Simmered	3½ oz.	100	165	1480

Organ Meats	Serving size	Weight (grams)	Calories (Kcal)	Phenylalanine (mg.)
Lamb Liver, Broiled	3½ oz.	100	261	1268
Pork				
Bacon, Canadian, Broiled/Fried	1 slice	21	65	237
Bacon, Cured, Broiled/Fried Crisp	3 strips	23	147	258
Blade, Lean Only	2 slices	61	134	740
Ham, Fresh, Lean Only	2 slices	75	167	1141
Ham, Cured Butt, Lean Only	2 slices	64	102	677
Loin Chops, Lean Only	1 chop	68	170	925
Picnic Shoulder, Lean Only, Roasted	2 slices	45	81	516
Tenderloin, Lean Only, Roasted	3½ oz.	100	239	1208
Turkey				
All Classes, Flesh and Skin Roasted	3½ oz.	100	223	1287
All Classes, Flesh Only, Raw	3½ oz.	100	162	960
Veal				
Blade, Lean Only	1 steak	108	228	1460
Cutlet, Round, Lean Only	1 slice	70	194	1144
Loin Chop, Lean Only	1 med. chop	72	149	998

Veal	Serving size	Weight (grams)	Calories (Kcal)	Phenylalanine (mg.)
Sirloin, Lean Only, Roasted	2 slices	59	90	700
Sirloin Steak, Lean Only	½ steak	68	139	964
Vegetables				
Beans, Common White, Cooked	½ cup	100	118	429
Beans, Red Kidney, Cooked	2/5 cup	100	118	429
Beans, Lima, Cooked	⅝ cup	100	111	448
Beans, Lima, Cooked, Baked	⅝ cup	115	159	555
Bean Sprouts, Mung, Cooked	1 cup	100	28	154
Broccoli, Cooked	1 lg. stalk	100	26	112
Brussels sprouts, Cooked	⅔ cup, 6–7 sprouts	100	32	139
Corn, Sweet, Raw	1 med. ear	100	96	196
Kale, Cooked, No Stems	¾ cup	100	39	184
Lentils, Cooked, Drained	⅔ cup	100	106	359
Peas, Cooked	⅔ cup	100	71	211
Split Peas, Cooked	3½ oz.	100	115	400
Potato, Baked without Skin	1:3½" dia.	150	139	172
Soybeans, Mature, Cooked	½ cup	100	130	594
Spinach, Cooked	½ cup	90	21	116
Nuts and Seeds				
Almonds, Roasted and Salted	1 oz.	28	176	321

Nuts and Seeds	Serving size	Weight (grams)	Calories (Kcal)	Phenylalanine (mg.)
Cashews, Roasted	20–26 nuts	50	280	438
Peanuts, Roasted with Skin	3½ oz.	100	572	1534
Peanut Butter	1 Tbsp.	15	86	227
Pumpkin and Squash Kernels	3½ oz.	100	553	1624
Sunflower Seed Kernels	3½ oz.	100	560	1272
Soups				
Asparagus, Cream of, Canned, with Milk	1 serving	198	88	236
Bean with Bacon, Canned, made with Water	1 serving	207	145	369
Black Bean, Condensed, made with Water	1 serving	207	87	260
Clam Chowder, New England, Frozen, made with Milk	1 serving	196	173	321
Mushroom, Cream of, Condensed, made with Milk	1 serving	198	149	246
Oyster Stew, Frozen, made with Milk	1 serving	193	133	414
Pea, Green, made with Water	1 serving	204	113	287

Appendix 1

TREATING AN OVERDOSE

THE "CAINE" REACTION

Phase	Central Nervous System	Circulatory System	Respiratory System
Early stimulation	Excitement, apprehension; other symptoms of emotional instability. Sudden headache. Nausea, vomiting. "Twitchings" of muscles, particularly of face, fingers.	Pulse varies; probably will slow. (Usual) elevation in blood pressure. Fall in blood pressure may occur. Pallor of skin.	Increased respiratory rate *and* depth.
Advanced stimulation	Convulsions (tonic and clonic—) resembles Grand Mal Seizure.	Increase in both pulse rate *and* blood pressure.	Cyanosis, dyspnea. Rapid (gasping or irregular) respiration.

Phase	Central Nervous System	Circulatory System	Respiratory System
Depression	Paralysis of muscles. Loss of reflexes. Unconsciousness. Loss of vital functions. Death.	Circulatory failure. No palpable pulse. Death.	Respiratory failure. Ashen gray cyanosis. Death.

TREATMENT OF THE "CAINE" REACTION

1. Administration of oxygen; by positive pressure and artificial respiration if necessary.
2. Trendelenburg position (head down). Wrap arms and legs if necessary to increase central return of blood.
3. Inject small amounts of short-acting barbiturates (e.g., 25–50 mg. Sodium Pentothal), *if* convulsions are present. May be repeated but *gently.* Do *not* force general effect to point of no return.
4. Administer intravenous stimulants for cardiotonic affect (e.g., phenylephrine 10–20 mg.).
5. Keep patient cool, and keep crowds away.
6. General muscle relaxants may be given (e.g., curare, succinylcholine) to facilitate administration of positive pressure oxygen.
7. Continuously monitor vital signs.

Appendix 2

THE COFFEE ENEMA

REASON: Coffee contains three related alkaloid substances: caffeine, theophylline, and theobromine. These alkaloids stimulate the CNS (central nervous system), act on the kidneys to produce diuresis (urination), stimulate the heart muscle, and relax the smooth muscles (such as the bronchi).

Caffeine is also a colon and liver stimulant. The liver (the largest organ in the body) detoxifies harmful substances and can, over a period of years, become "swamped". During a coffee enema some of the coffee is absorbed into the portal blood system from the colon. The portal system veins go to the liver where the coffee stimulates the liver to "flush out" the bile. In this manner the coffee enema aids the liver in the process of detoxifying the body.

You may wonder why you cannot merely drink coffee and achieve the same results as a coffee enema. Drinking coffee *is* more convenient, however, (1) absorption by this route is less effective; (2) when coffee is drunk it goes through chemical changes in the stomach which are not beneficial to the system and can slow down the flow of bile.

However, an occasional cup (150–250 mg. of caffeine in 1–2 cups of coffee or tea) is useful in certain situations. Taking 500 mg. of caffeine may increase the basal metabolic rate as much as 10–25% for approximately one to three hours after ingestion.

INDICATIONS FOR USE: It is advisable to use coffee enemas during cleansing reactions. Symptoms of a cleansing reaction can include headache, nausea, indigestion, irritability, and muscle pain. They can also be used in the case of cold or flu symptoms, hepatitis, or mononucleosis.

FREQUENCY: As a general cleansing program enemas can be used two times a week for four weeks, and then once every three months. If you are fasting, frequency is one or two enemas per day, particularly if you are feeling "toxic". If you are experiencing a cleansing reaction frequency can be from once a day to every few hours for a few days.

TOXICITY: Scare stories describing deaths due to coffee enemas have been printed in some newspaper and journal articles. In these cases patients were taking over ten to twelve coffee enemas per day for prolonged periods of time. This is indeed toxic.

As long as the frequency stays within these guidelines we have had no serious problems. Occasionally, the coffee causes too much stimulation or abdominal discomfort and should be replaced by

1 lemon (squeezed) and 2 cloves of garlic (pressed to oil) in 2 quarts of water

or

1 part buttermilk to 2 parts water

or

Equal parts camomile and catnip tea

Children may be given smaller amounts of coffee solution for earaches, colds, coughs, flu, etc., with great results. Dosages should be:

Infants	50–100cc
3–6	1 pint
6–12	1 quart
12 and older	1–2 quarts

TIME: Allow thirty to sixty minutes from start to finish.

PREPARATION OF THE COFFEE ENEMA SOLUTION

Using a good quality coffee (Columbian, Kava, Yuban; not decaffeinated or instant, which have too many chemicals) select one of the following methods.

A. 1. Boil approximately 2–3 heaping tablespoons of ground coffee per quart of water for 5 minutes, and then simmer for 10 minutes. You will need 2 quarts.
   2. Cool the liquid coffee by immersing the pot of coffee in a sink full of cold water and stirring the coffee and the water. Cool the coffee to the point at which the elbow feels neither hot nor cold when immersed in it. Strain grounds from the coffee.
   3. Pour the coffee into the enema bag.

This method is a little faster:

B. 1. Boil approximately 4 heaping tablespoons of ground coffee in 2 cups of water for 10 minutes.

2. Dilute the coffee with enough cold water to make up the 1½ to 2 quarts of solution.
3. Check the temperature with your elbow as in Method A, Step 2. Adjust as necessary.
4. Pour the coffee into the enema bag.

C. 1. Dilute ¾ to 1 cup of coffee concentrate* with 5 to 7 cups of water. This will make a coffee solution comparable in strength to that obtained by following Method A or B.
2. Heat the liquid coffee to a tepid temperature. Check the temperature as in Method A, Step 2.
3. Pour the coffee into the enema bag.

ADMINISTERING THE ENEMA

The best time of the day to do a coffee enema is in the morning after you have had at least one bowel movement. Some people also find it useful in helping them to go to sleep at night.

Pour the coffee solution into the enema bag.

Place the enema bag so that it will hang 2 feet above the rectum when you lie down on your side. Do not hang the bag too high as you do not want too

**The concentrate is made using a "Toddy Maker" which is available at many coffee and tea supply shops for about $16.00. One pound of ground coffee is soaked for 12 to 24 hours in two quarts of water and then filtered. This is based on a Peruvian method and results in a less acidic coffee.*

The coffee concentrate which is not used within one or two weeks should be frozen in separate, one cup containers and thawed out as needed for use.

much gravity pressure. If one lies on a slant board while taking the enema, the solution will reach further into the colon.

Release a little coffee solution from the bag so there is no air in the tubing.

Lubricate the tip of the enema nozzle and your rectum with oil (coconut, sesame, Wonder Balm, etc.).

Insert the tip of the nozzle into the rectum slowly. To help relax the rectal sphincter muscle, do slow and deep, or rapid and shallow breathing. You may then:

> release the coffee from the enema bag in one slow, continuous flow

OR

> decrease the volume of coffee entering by pinching the metal pinch valve on the tubing with your thumb and forefinger

OR

> allow approximately ½ cup of coffee in at a time, pinching off the tubing in between and taking a few deep breaths to help your colon relax any tensions.

If you experience any discomfort, such as cramping, pinch off the tubing and continue with slow, deep breathing until the cramping stops.

After all of the coffee has been inserted lie on your back with your knees slightly bent for about 2 minutes.

Alternate lying on the right and left side, or you may do the entire enema on your right or left side. Shoulder stands or head stand for up to 3 minutes are fine if you have been taught how to do them safely.

Retain the coffee for 10 to 12 minutes, if possible.

A shorter retention time is therapeutic, but longer retention time is better.

Release the enema.

A feeling of "well-being" is common after the enema. If you are uncomfortably "speedy" or hyperirritable, you may try reducing the amount of coffee to water, or use one of the other enema solutions previously mentioned.

Appendix 3

ADULTERANTS IN COCAINE

The substances used to "cut" or dilute the more expensive cocaine are grouped in three categories:

1. *Anesthetic Cut:* substances producing the *numbing effect* of cocaine and which give similar sensations.
2. *Active Cut:* substances that have some of the *stimulating* or *mood* altering properties of cocaine.
3. *Inert Cut:* substances that look like cocaine but offer no effects. Adding nothing to the cocaine "high", they are simply white powders or crystals used to cut the drug.

Anesthetic Cuts

Procaine: also known as novocain, allocaine, biocaine, clinocaine, ethocaine, genocaine, and syncaine. It is synthetic and structurally related to cocaine. A rapid acting local anesthetic of short duration that imparts some of the numbing effects of cocaine. It affects both sensory and motor nerves. This is a relatively safe cut. Freebase procaine is sometimes used as a cocaine cut which occurs as a dull white powder. Poorly soluble in water and therefore tends to linger in the nose and sometimes causes sneezing.

Tetracaine: has same anesthetic potency as cocaine. Anesthetic effect lasts longer than procaine. Toxicity is 7 times that of procaine, and 2–3 times that of cocaine.

Benzocaine: very low toxicity and considered safe for inhalation and ingestion. Poor water solubility which makes it dangerous if injected. Can form blood clots, emboli, and other complications. Common street adulterant.

Butacaine: another synthetic related to cocaine. It comes as a dullish white powder. Swift numbing effect and some of the stimulating properties of cocaine. More toxic than cocaine and more irritating to the mucous membranes. May cause nosebleeds.

Lidocaine: also known as lignocaine and xylocaine. Responds to the bleach test. Same toxicity as cocaine. Occurs as an odorless, white crystalline powder with a slightly bitter taste.

Active Cuts

Methedrine: like all amphetamine derivatives this is a powerful stimulant of the central nervous system, sympathetic nervous system, and cerebral center. It is an odorless, bitter tasting, fine white crystal or crystalline powder. Side effects are very much like cocaine, although it will also cause tight feeling in the neck and facial muscles (especially the jaw), sharp bitter taste, and intense pain in the nose when snorted. Tolerance to methedrine can develop, and paranoia is often the by-product of extended and excessive use.

Pemoline: a synthetic stimulant. Fine shiny, white crystalline powder with a silky, almost greasy feeling to the touch when rubbed between the fingers. Imitates cocaine stimulation very well. Lengthens the duration of the cocaine "high" by 3–4 times. Pemoline is tasteless and causes no irritation to the nose. There is no law against Pemoline but the government has issued directives that it be sold only to legal organizations.

PCP: commonly called angel dust. While the precise pharmacological mechanisms are not completely understood, this is known to be a dangerous cut which should be avoided. It is thought to cause brain cell damage with lingering side effects.

Yohimbine, (aphrodine, corynine): this cut is thought to have psychoactive and aphrodisiac properties. Derived from the plant *(coryanthe yohimbe),* it is usually a dull fluffy white powder, sometimes with a yellowish tinge, and is tasteless. It may act as an aphrodisiac by inhibiting serotonin levels in the brain, by stimulating the spinal ganglia which affect erection, and by bringing increased blood to the genital zone. The warm shivers experienced under yohimbine are enjoyable during intercourse and may give the illusion of bodies melting into one another. Yohimbine does not combine well with other drugs when used as a cut in cocaine, especially amphetamines. *Can produce a violent reaction if one uses cocaine cut with yohimbine and begins drinking alcohol.* Yohimbine is legal, but the recent DEA directive has made it difficult to obtain from chemical supply houses.

Inert Cuts

Mannite: white powder. Slightly sweet taste. Available in 3 forms: powder, granules and compressed blocks. Preferred form is the block. Sold in Europe as a baby laxative. Has good cocaine-like appearance. Rapidly absorbed by the mucous membranes. Taste barely noticeable when mixed. Non-toxic, non-irritating. May cause slight post-nasal drip. May cause laxative effect. Will pass flame test.

Inositol: this is a B vitamin and non-toxic. White crystalline granular with slightly sweet taste. Sparkling appearance. Absorbs well on mucous membranes.

Lactose: white crystalline powder. Odorless and slightly sweet taste. Non-toxic. Will absorb moisture. Causes sneezing.

Talc: soft, finely powdered mineral. Possibly cancer causing owing to the asbestos it contains. Insoluble in water. Dangerous to inject—can cause emboli or blood clots.

Cornstarch: same as talc; not carcinogenic.

Quinine: odorless, bitter tasting white crystalline powder. Very toxic side effects—ringing in the ears, headaches, impaired hearing, nausea, diarrhea, visual disturbances, and vertigo. Very dangerous to inject.

Miscellaneous Cuts

There are several other adulterants (cuts) worth mentioning. Occasionally they are used to cut cocaine. The list would include boric acid, epsom salts (this is generally processed by dealers before using and after processing it would probably best be grouped under inert cuts as it will add bulk without taste). Richard Rhodes in the January 1975 article *A Very Expensive High* made mention of the use of an *amino acid* as a cocaine adulterant. As is true with all amino acids, it would add bulk without taste and therefore fall under the category of an inert cut.

Another relatively harmless cut is caffeine. Due to the fact that the required dosage is so high to produce a bodily effect, caffeine will mainly dilute the product. Ephedrine Sulfate, a stimulant derived from the oriental Ephedra plant is also used as an adulterant due to the fact that it is a sympathetic nervous system stimulant and moderately central nervous system stimulant with effects lasting 2-4 hours. It is generally safe. Dealers have also been known to use *aspirin* and *flour* as cocaine cuts. Both are relatively harmless as cocaine adulterants.

Appendix 4

BARTKO'S BRAIN HYPOXIA STUDIES*

CONCLUSIONS

Changes in oxygen balance and glucose metabolism have been followed in arterial and venous blood of the brain, in cerebrospinal fluid, and in the peripheral region under study, together with changes of certain metabolites of the energy metabolism (glycogen, lactate, ATP, ADP, ATP/ADP, AMP, certain amino acids) in the cerebral cortex of dogs under conditions of an experimental selective brain hypoxia.

1. The arteriovenous difference in the *oxygen volume* of the brain increased in a significant degree; in view of the *unchanging oxygen concentration* of the arterial blood *this speaks for its substantially improved utilization.* The improved oxygen utilization

**Quoted from Bartko (1971). See this important work for more results re: oxygen balance, particularly "oxygen offer" values.*

became manifest in the *increase* of the *coefficient of its utilization.* The *oxygen consumption* and *oxygen offer decreased.*

2. At the periphery a significant decrease occurred only in oxygen consumption. All the remaining parameters fluctuated around the initial values.

3. The arterial glycemia level rose by more than 50%; glucose concentration in the venous blood of the brain rose also, but to a lesser degree and the increase in the arteriovenous glucose difference was 2–3 times higher than the starting values. Glucose offer and consumption in the brain were significantly lowered. Rise of the glucose concentration in the cerebrospinal fluid lagged behind that in the arterial and venous glycemia and was higher than in the control group, which testifies to a *higher permeability of the blood-liquor barrier by sugars.*

4. There exists a significant correlation between a decreased glucose consumption and a rise in the arteriovenous glucose difference and also an increased percentual glucose extraction. A comparison of the percentual oxygen utilization with the percentual glucose extraction has shown that the trend of their increase in the first hour of selective brain hypoxia is similar (+85.75 and +79.73%, respectively); during the second hour, oxygen utilization went on to increase until it was twice the starting value (+102.20% increase), while the percentual glucose extraction, even though higher than the initial value, nevertheless decreased (+24.28%).

5. The *content* of *lactic acid* in the *cerebral cortex increased* by 254.96–552.50% in comparison with the initial value which is *proof* of an *intensive anaerobic glycolysis. Glycogen and ATP contents* (including the ratio ATP/ADP and Σ ATP+ADP+AMP),

on the contrary, *remained relatively stable* during the first hour of brain hypoxia. A significant decline was observed only in the second hour. The AMP content rose significantly along with an unchanging APD level.

6. Changes in the levels of *some amino acids* speak for their participation in the energy metabolism of the brain in the course of selective brain hypoxia. After 1 hour of hypoxia we observed a significant increase in *glutamic and gamma-aminobutyric acid contents,* but these values returned to normal levels after 2 hours of brain hypoxia.

7. A slowing of the frequency waves was observed in the EEG picture, with the appearance of theta and delta activity, and a subsequent depression in amplitude.

REFERENCES

ALPERS, D.H., SOLIN, M. AND INSELBACHER, K.J., 1968. "Role of Lipid Peroxidation in the Pathogenesis of Carbon Tetrachloride-Induced Liver Injury." *Mol Pharmacol* 4, 566.

BACHELARD, H.S., 1981. *Brain Biochemistry,* 2nd Ed. Chapman and Hall, London.

BARCHAS, J.D., et al. (Eds.), 1977. *Psychopharmacology.* Oxford University, New York.

BARDSLEY, M.E. AND BACHELARD, H.S., 1981. "Catecholamine Levels and Tyrosine Hydroxylase Activity in Rat Brain Regions After Chronic Treatment, and Withdrawal of, Methamphetamine." *Biochem. Pharmac.,* in press.

BARTKO, D., 1971. *Experimental Brain Hypoxia.* University Park Press, Baltimore.

BENAKIS, A. AND THOMASSET, M., 1969. "Metabolism of Amphetamines and Their Interaction With Other Drugs" in *Abuse of Central Stimulants* (ed. Sjoqvist, A. and Tottie, M.), Almqvist and Wiksell, Stockholm, pp. 409–434.

BOGERT, L.J., BRIGGS, G.M., AND CALLOWAY, D.H., 1979. *Nutrition and Physical Fitness.* 10th ed. Philadelphia: Saunders.

BORISON, et al. "Metabolism of the Antidepressant Amino Acid, L-Phenylalanine." FASEB Meeting, Atlantic City, N.J., April 9–14, 1978.

CAHILL, G.F., 1978. "Famine Symposium—Physiology of Acute Starvation in Man." *Ecology of Food and Nutrition* 6:221–230.

CAMERON, E. AND PAULING, L., 1979. *Cancer and Vitamin C.* Menlo Park, California: Linus Pauling Institute.

CHERASKIN, E., RINGSDORF, W.M., AND CLARK, J.W., 1968. *Diet and Disease.* New Canaan, Connecticut: Keats Publishing Company.

CHIU-NAN LAI, 1978. "Chlorophyll: The Active Factor in Wheat Sprout Extract Inhibiting the Metabolic Activation of Carcinogens in Vitro." *Nutrition and Cancer I* (3).

CLEAVE, T. AND CAMPBELL, G., 1966. *Diabetes, Coronary Thrombosis and the Saccharine Disease.* Wright and Sons, Publishers.

COLOMBETTI, G. AND MONTI, S., 1971. Eur. Bio-phys. Congr., Proc., 1st. 2:45–53.

CUTTING, W.C., 1969. *Handbook of Pharmacology,* 4th Ed. Meredith, New York.

DENBER, H.C.B. (Ed.), 1975. *Psychopharmacological Treatment.* Dekker, New York.

ELWOOD, C., 1965. *Feel Like A Million,* 46, Pocket Books.

FREDERICKS, C. AND BAILEY, H., 1965. *Food Facts and Fallacies.* New York: Galahad Books.

FREDERICKS, C. AND GOODMAN, H., 1969. *Low Blood Sugar and You.* New York: Grosset & Dunlap.

FREDERICKS, C., 1976. *Psycho-Nutrition.* Grosset & Dunlap, New York.

FRUTON, JOSEPH AND SIMMONDS, SOFIA, 1958. p. 792, *General Biochemistry,* 2nd Ed.; Wiley.

GELENBERG, A., May 1980. *Tyrosine For the Treatment of Depression. American J. Psy.,* 147–622.

GOLBERG, L., 1982. "New Directions in Food Toxicology." *Chem Ind. 11, 355.*

GOLDBERG, I., August 1980. *Tyrosine in Depression.* Lancet, 364.

GOODHART, R.S. AND SHILS, M.E., 1980. *Modern Nutrition in Health and Disease,* 5th Ed., Philadelphia: Lea & Febiger.

GOODMAN, L.S. & GILMAN, A., 1970. *The Pharmacological Basis of Therapeutics,* 4th Ed. Macmillan, New York.

CROWDON, A., *Neurotransmitter Precursors in the Diet.* In "Nutrition and the Brain," Wurtman and Wurtman, Eds., 117–181, Raven Press, 1979.

HARPER, HAROLD, *Review of Physiological Chemistry,* 12th Ed., p. 357, Lange Med. Publ, 1969.

HOFFER, A., *Orthomolecular Psychiatry.* D. Hawkins and L. Pauling (Eds.). Freeman & Co., San Francisco, p. 238, 1973.

HORROBIN, D.F., et al., 1979. "The Nutritional Regulation of T Lymphocyte Function." *Medical Hypotheses* 5:969–985.

HUGHES, R.E., 1981. *Vitamin C, Some Current Problems.* London: British Nutrition Foundation, p. 27.

JAFFE, W.G., 1973. "Toxic Proteins and Peptides." In: NAS.

JOHNSON, F.C., 1979. "The Antioxidant Vitamins." *CRC Crit Rev. Food Sci Nutr* 11:270.

JOHNSON, F.C., 1983. "Cancer Promoters and Initiators, and the Free Radical Theory of Carcinogenesis." *Nutr Cancer* 4, 169–170.

JOHNSON, F.C., 1982. "Carcinogenesis, Vascular Disease, and the Free Radical Reaction." *Nutr Cancer 3, 117–121.*

KUNIN, R.A., 1980. *Mega-Nutrition.* McGraw-Hill, New York.

LAPEDES, DANIEL. *Encyclopedia of Food, Agriculture and Nutrition.* p. 208. McGraw-Hill, 1977.

LESSER, M., 1980. *Nutrition and Vitamin Therapy.* Grove Press, New York.

LOVENBERG, W., 1973. "Some Vaso- and Psychoactive Substances in Food: Amines, Stimulants, Depressants and Hallucinogens." In: NAS.

LUNDBERG, W.O., 1961. *Autoxidation & Antioxidants.* Wiley-Interscience, New York.

MANDELL, A.J. AND MORGAN, M., 1970. "Amphetamine Induced Increase in Tyrosine Hydroxylase Activity." *Nature,* 227, 75–76.

MANN, J.A., 1980. *Secrets of Life Extension.* Harbor Publishing, San Francisco.

MANNING, D.H., STRANG, R.H.C. AND BACHELARD, H.S., 1974. "Changes In Cerebral Carbohydrate Metabolism In the Rat After Acute and Chronic Treatment With, and Withdrawal of Methamphetamine." *Biochem. Pharmacol.* 23, 1205–1209.

MADRONES, J., 1960. "International Review of Neurobiology." C.C. Pfeiffer and J.R. Smythies (Eds.). Academic Press, New York, p. 41.

NATIONAL ACADEMY OF SCIENCES, 1973. *Toxicants Occurring Naturally in Foods.* Washington, D.C.

NEWBOLD, H.L., 1975. *Mega-Nutrients for Your Nerves.* Peter Wyden, New York.

PARDRIDGE, R., 1977. *Regulation of Amino Acid Availability to the Brain. In "Nutrition and the Brain,"* Wurtman and Wurtman, Eds., 141-204, Raven Press.

PAULING, L., 1978. "An Orthomolecular Physician." *Linus Pauling Institute Newsletter I* (4):1–3.

PENNINGTON, J. AND CHURCH, H.N., 1980. *Food Values of Portions Commonly Used.* J.B. Lippincott, Philadelphia.

PFEIFFER, C., 1975. *Mental & Elemental Nutrients.* Keats, New Canaan, Connecticut.

PHILPOTT, W. AND KHALEELUDDIN, K. Society for Clinical Ecology, 14th Annual Meeting, San Diego, CA, Oct. 28, 1979.

POST, R., 1975. *Cocaine Psychoses.* Am. J. Psychiatry, Vol. 132: 225–31.

RANBY, B. AND RABEK, J.F. (Eds.), 1978. *Singlet Oxygen.* Wiley-Interscience, New York.

RAVEL, J.M., FELSING, B., LANSFORD, E.M., TRUBEY, R.H. AND SHIVE, W., 1955. *Reversal of Alcohol Toxicity by Glutamine.* Vol. 214, No. 2., pp. 497–501.

ROE, D.A., 1976. *Drug-Induced Nutritional Deficiencies.* Westport, Connecticut: AVI Publishing.

ROGERS, L.L., PELTON, R.B., AND WILLIAMS, R., 1956. "Amino Acid Supplementation and Voluntary Alcohol Consumption by Rats." *The Journal of Biological Chemistry,* Vol. 220, No. 1, pp. 321–323.

ROGERS, L.L. AND PELTON, R.B., 1957. "Effect of Glutamine on IQ Scores of Mentally Deficient Children." *Texas Reports on Biology and Medicine,* Vol. 15, No. 1, pp. 84–90.

ROGERS, L.L., 1957. "Glutamine in the Treatment of Alcoholism." *Quarterly Journal of Studies on Alcohol 18*(4):581.

ROGERS, L.L., PELTON, R.B. AND WILLIAMS, R., 1955. "Voluntary Alcohol Consumption by Rats Following Administration of Glutamine." Vol. 214, No. 2, pp. 503–506.

ROSENFELD, I. AND BEATH, O., 1964. *Selenium: Geobotany, Biochemistry, Toxicity and Nutrition.* New York: Academic Press.

RUDOLPH, C., JR., 1977. "Trace Element Patterning in Degenerative Diseases." *Journal of the International Academy of Preventive Medicine.*

SCHAUSS, A., 1981. *Diet, Crime & Delinquency.* Parker House, Berkeley, California.

SHALITA, B. AND DIKSTEIN, S., 1979. *Tyrosine Prevents Hypertension in DOCA-Saline Treated Uninephrectomized Rats.* Pflugers Archive, 379:245.

SHAMBERGER, R.J. AND FROST, D.V.C., 1969. "Possible Protective Effect of Selenium Against Human Cancer." *Canadian Medical Association Journal 100:*682.

SHIVE, W., et al., 1957. "Glutamine in Treatment of Peptic Ulcer." *Texas State Journal of Medicine 53:*840.

SIEGEL, R.K., 1982. *Cocaine Smoking.* J. Psychoactive Drugs, Vol. 14 (4): 271–359.

SIMIC, M.G. & KAREL, M., 1980. *Autoxidation in Food and Biological Systems.* Plenum, New York.

STEIN, et al., 1975. *Memory Enhancement by Central Administration of Norepinephrine.* Brain Res., 84: 329–335.

UTENA, H., EZOE, T., KATO, N. AND HADA, H., 1959. "Effects of Chronic Administration of Methamphetamine in Enzymic Patterns in Brain Tissue." *J. Neurochem.* 4, 161–169.

VAN DYKE, C. AND BYCK, R., 1982. "Cocaine." *Scientific American* Vol. 246(3): 128–141.

WEINER, M.A., 1981. *The Way of the Skeptical Nutritionist.* Macmillan, New York.

WEINER, M.A., 1980. *Weiner's Herbal.* Stein & Day, New York.

WHEELER, J.I. AND TRUNNEL, J.B. "Preliminary Report on Experiments With Orally Administered Glutamine in Treatment of Alcoholics." ACS. Houston, December, 1955.

WHITE, ABRAHAM, et al, 1978. *Principles of Biochemistry,* 6th Ed., p. 732. McGraw-Hill.

WILLIAMS, R.J. "Alcoholism: The Nutritional Approach." University of Texas Press, Austin (1959), p. 100.

WILLIAMS, R.J. AND LANDSFORD, E.M. "The Encyclopedia of Biochemistry." Reinhold. New York, (1959) p. 375.

WILLIAMS, R.J., 1973. *Nutrition Against Disease.* New York: Bantam.

YOSHIDA, O., BROWN, R.R., AND BRYAN, G.T., 1971. "A Possible Role of Urinary Metabolites of Tryptophan in the Heterotropic Recurrence of Bladder Cancer in Man." *American Journal of Clinical Nutrition 24:*848.